NEW DEVELOPMENTS IN MEDICAL RESEARCH

INTEGRATIVE MEDICINE

ITS ROLE FOR OUR FUTURE MEDICINE

New Developments in Medical Research

Additional books in this series can be found on Nova's website under the Series tab.

Additional e-books in this series can be found on Nova's website under the e-book tab.

Health Care in Transition

Additional books in this series can be found on Nova's website under the Series tab.

Additional e-books in this series can be found on Nova's website under the e-book tab.

NEW DEVELOPMENTS IN MEDICAL RESEARCH

INTEGRATIVE MEDICINE

ITS ROLE FOR OUR FUTURE MEDICINE

TOKU TAKAHASHI

NOVA BIOMEDICAL

New York

For permission to use material from this book please contact us:
Telephone 631-231-7269; Fax 631-231-8175
Web Site: http://www.novapublishers.com

NOTICE TO THE READER

Additional color graphics may be available in the e-book version of this book.

Library of Congress Cataloging-in-Publication Data

ISBN: 978-1-62618-543-2

Library of Congress Control Number: 2013935907

Published by Nova Science Publishers, Inc. † New York

This book is dedicated to my family:
Ikuyo, Junko, Tomoko, Ryota, Kota, Daisuke, Reiko, Eisuke and Haru.

To my mother, wife, children and grandchildren – for their support, encouragement and love.

CONTENTS

PREFACE

Conventional Western medicine (CWM) has made a great contribution to our health and well-being in the last several decades. However, CWM pays less attention to self-healing, mind-body interactions, preventive medicine, and doctor-patient relationship. Complementary and alternative medicine (CAM) is a diverse group of health care systems, practices, and products that are not presently considered a part of CWM. The interest in CAM has increased dramatically over the past decade. Mind-body techniques considered as CAM are meditation, Yoga, Tai-chi, Qi-gong, and music therapy. Manual and manipulative methods in CAM include chiropractic, massage, acupuncture, and touch therapy.

There is a great deal of research and evidence supporting CAM therapies. The beneficial effects of CAM are mainly due to reduction of stress responses and pain pathways. Meditation, Yoga, Tai-chi, Qi-gong, and music therapy promote these effects mainly via stimulation of brain activity and its networking (top-down pathway), while chiropractic, massage, acupuncture, and touch therapy promote these effects mainly via stimulation of peripheral sensory nerves (bottom-up pathway).

Both pathways stimulate the release of various substances in the brain, such as opioid and oxytocin, which mediate anti-stress and analgesic effects. Thus, it is possible to treat physical diseases through the central and peripheral nervous system. Once these CAM therapies are proven to be safe and effective, CAM will become adopted into conventional health care as new approaches to health care emerge.

Integrative medicine combines mainstream medical therapies (CWM) and certain CAM therapies for which there is some high-quality scientific evidence of safety and effectiveness. Integrative medicine can cover the current problems of CWM by integrating the efficacy of both CWM and CAM. Future medicine should pay great attention to all aspects of a person's lifestyle. The integrative medicine approach emphasizes the innate healing mechanism of the human being. We can change the medical system by educating CWM doctors and CAM practitioners on the integrative medicine approach. We also need to educate the public so they may take greater responsibility for their health.

ACKNOWLEDGEMENTS

The author wishes to thank the following for their fruitful collaboration.

From University of Michigan

Drs. Kazumi Nakamura, Susumu Kurosawa, Kenji Hosoda, Yuichiro Kojima, Yasuhiro Tsunoda, Mayumi Taniuchi, Chun Hsu, Koji Nakao, Yohei Mizuta, Ali Yazdani, Tadashi Ishiguchi, Bill Hasler, John Wiley, and Chung Owyang.

From Duke University

Drs. Hitoshi Tada, Mikio Fujita, Toru Kono, Akiko Shiotani, Sebastian G. de la Fuente, Kenichiro Uemura, Makoto Tatewaki, Tomio Ueno, Jose Balestrini, Woo Yong Lee, Masahiro Iwa, Hiroyuki Fukuda, Daisuke Tsuchida, Yukiomi Nakade, Kiyoshi Tsukamoto, Constant Masere, Hajime Ariga, Kenji Imai, Erito Mochiki, Chris Mantyh, and Theodore Pappas.

From Medical College of Wisconsin

Drs. Hitoshi Nakajima, Weidong Tong, Jun Zheng, Mehmet Bulbul, Koichi Kamiyama, Aaron Zietlow, Anthony Dobner, Tim Ridolfi, Hiroshi Taniguchi, Sazu Yoshimoto, Diana Cerjak, Jung-Myun Kwak, Jonathan Ramprasad, Irena Gribovskaja-Rupp, Reji Babygirija, Kirk Ludwig, and Thomas Chelimsky.

LIST OF ABBREVIATIONS

A

adrenocorticotropic hormone (ACTH)
alpha-linolenic acid (ALA)
American Academy of Medical Acupuncture (AAMA)
American massage therapy association (AMTA)
anterior cingulate cortex (ACC)
arachidonic acid (AA)
atrial natriuretic peptide (ANP)

B

blood brain barrier (BBB)
body mass index (BMI)
brain derived neurotrophic factor (BDNF)

C

cerebrospinal fluid (CSF)
central nervous system (CNS)
chemoreceptor trigger zone (CTZ)
complementary and alternative medicine (CAM)
conventional Western medicine (CWM)
corticotropin releasing factor (CRF)
cyclo-oxygenase (COX)
cytochrome P450 (CYP)

D

docosahexaenoic acid (DHA)
dopamine (DA)
dorsal motor nucleus of vagi (DMV)
dorsal vagal complex (DVC)

E

eicosapentaenoic acid (EPA)
electroacupuncture (EA)
electrocardiography (ECG)
electroencephalography (EEG)
evidence-based medicine (EBM)
endothelial nitric oxide synthase (eNOS)

F

focused attention (FA)
functional dyspepsia (FD)
functional magnetic resonance imaging (fMRI)

G

gastrointestinal (GI)
gamma-aminobutyric acid (GABA)

H

heart rate variability (HRV)
high frequency (HF)
hypothalamic-pituitary-adrenal (HPA)

I

irritable bowel syndrome (IBS)
integrative mind body training (IBMT)

L

long-term potentiation (LTP)
loving-kindness meditation (LKM)
low frequency (LF)

M

maternal-fetal attachment scale (MFAS)
3,4 methylenedioxymethamphetamine (MDMA)
mindfulness-based stress reduction (MBSR)
mindfulness-based cognitive therapy (MBCT)

N

nitric oxide (NO)
non-steroidal anti-inflammatory drugs (NSAIDs)
nucleus tractus solitarius (NTS)

O

open monitoring (OM)
oxytocin (OXT)
oxytocin knockout mice (OXT-KO)

P

paraventricular nucleus (PVN)
pericardium-6 (PC6)
periaqueductal gray (PAG)
positron emission tomography (PET)
posterior cingulate cortex (PCC)
post-traumatic stress disorders (PTSD)
proton pump inhibitors (PPIs)
prefrontal cortex (PFC)
prostaglandins (PG)

R

randomized controlled trials (RCTs)
rostral ventrolateral medulla (RVLM)

S

social anxiety disorder (SAD)
stomach-25 (ST-25)
stomach-36 (ST-36)
selective serotonin reuptake inhibitors (SSRIs)
supraoptic nucleus (SON)

T

transcutaneous electrical nerve stimulation (TENS)
traditional Chinese medicine (TCM)

Chapter 1

COMPLEMENTARY AND ALTERNATIVE MEDICINE (CAM)

Complementary and alternative medicine (CAM) is a group of diverse medical and health care systems, practices, and products that are not presently considered a part of conventional Western medicine (CWM). While it is true that CWM has established an ever-growing expansion of scientific knowledge, basic science research, and technology, it is also true that interest in CAM has increased dramatically over the past decade.

Mind-body medicine uses variety of techniques designed to enhance the mind's capacity to affect bodily function and symptoms. The techniques considered as CAM are meditation, Yoga, Tai chi, Qi-gong, and music therapy. Manual and manipulative methods in CAM include chiropractic, massage, acupuncture, and touch therapy.

While some scientific evidence exists regarding some CAM therapies, for most there are key questions that have yet to be answered through well-designed scientific studies. For example, "Do these therapies work for the diseases or medical conditions for which they are designed?", "Are the therapies proven to be safe?"

Once those therapies are proven to be safe and effective, CAM will become adopted into conventional health care as new approaches to health care emerge.

1. Wide Spread Use of CAM

Lifetime prevalence of CAM therapy use in the US has increased steadily since 1950. In fact, recent studies have shown that CAM has increasingly been accepted in the US (Barnes et al., 2004) and Europe (Fisher et al., 1994). In 1999, approximately 30% of respondents were reported for using at least one form of CAM (Frass et al., 2012).

Although these numbers have been increasing in recent years, the debate about the clinical effectiveness of unconventional methods has been controversial among many medical professionals. However, the attitude of the general population toward CAM is generally positive. Although few scientific data exist for much of the discipline, CAM has evolved into a successful, commercially available business throughout the world. Additionally, journals focused on CAM, along with recent basic and clinical science research, have improved the understanding of the benefits gained from these various therapies and modalities.

In most countries, CAM is not covered by national insurance systems, and users pay almost all costs out of their pockets. This willingness to pay reflects the public's general acceptance of CAM and also suggests that CAM therapies have benefits that outweigh their costs. The estimated expenditures for alternative medicine professional services increased by 45% between 1990 and 1997 and were conservatively estimated at $21 billion in 1997, with at least $12 billion paid out of pocket. This amount exceeded the 1997 out-of-pocket expenditures for all hospitalizations in the US. A national health survey in 2007 revealed that more than $34 billion was spent on CAM annually in the US. In Germany, where some forms of CAM are covered by insurance, costs for alternative therapies in 2000 accounted for about one-tenth of expenditures on general medical treatments (Eisenberg, 1997; Eisenberg et al., 1998).

The clinical effectiveness of CAM has been controversial. Frass et al. (2012) conducted a systematic search of the existing literature utilizing different databases to research the use and acceptance of CAM among the general population and medical personnel. Prevalence rates of CAM in each of the included studies were between 5% and 75%. The data demonstrated that chiropractic manipulation, herbal medicine, massage, and homeopathy were the therapies most commonly used by the general population. Most of the users were women, middle aged, and well educated. The ailments most often associated with CAM utilization included back pain, depression, insomnia, severe headache or migraine, and stomach or intestinal illnesses (Frass et al., 2012).

2. CURRENT CIRCUMSTANCES OF CAM

Certainly, the gap between CWM and CAM is very substantive. It pertains to methodology and rigorous applications of scientific standards of evidence as well as to the meaning and context of illness and health.

2.1. The Lack of a Common Language between CAM and CWM

> "They are one people and have one language, and nothing will be with held from them which they purpose to do." So God said, "Come, let us go down and confound their speech." And so God scattered them upon the face of the Earth, and confused their languages, and they left off building the city, which was called Babel "because God there confounded the language of all the Earth" (Genesis 11:5–8).

Capsi et al. (2000) called the *Tower of Babel* as a metaphor to advocate dialogue as a way to bridge that gap between CAM and CWM. The most commonly addressed aspects of CAM in the medical literature are its safety, efficacy, and legislation. However, the different obstacles in the implementation of true health integration are unfortunately rarely addressed: the lack of a common language among CAM providers and CWM physicians.

For most CWM physicians, a genuine understanding of the underlying concepts and practices of CAM, such as acupuncture and homeopathy, is almost beyond achievement. This lack of understanding is not because physicians do not have the ability or willingness to understand CAM. The reason is that the CAM and CWM do not share the same language. The root of this discrepancy is directly related to the entire process of medical education of both CAM and CWM (Capsi et al. 2000).

According to traditional Chinese medicine (TCM) concepts, the energy force, known as *Qi* (pronounced *Chee*), runs through the body. *Qi* energy enters the body through specific acupuncture points and flows to deeper organ structures, bringing life-giving nourishment of a subtle energetic nature. Meridians are classified on the basis of the direction in which *Qi* flows on the surface of the body. If the flow of *Qi* is insufficient, or interrupted, *Yin* and *Yang* become unbalanced and illness may occur (Helms, 1998) (Figure 1.1). However, for most CWM physicians the words of *Qi*, meridians, and *Yin* and *Yang* cannot be understandable. Ahn et al. (2008) conducted a systematic review of studies directly evaluating the electrical characteristics of acupuncture structures and appropriate controls. There was no clear evidence to demonstrate the existence of acupuncture points or meridians (Ahn et al., 2008).

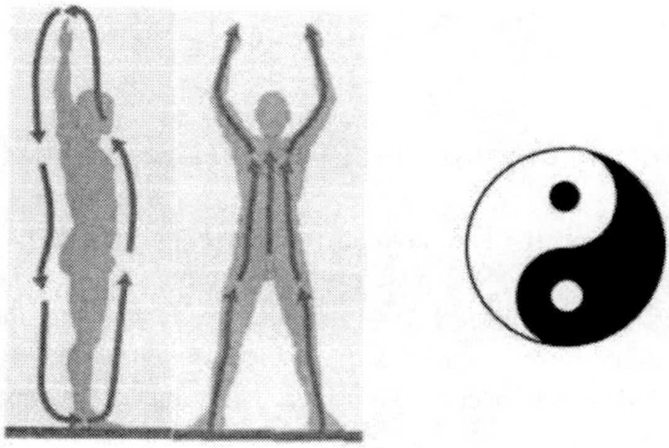

Figure 1.1. Flow of Qi (left) and symbol of Ying and Yan (right).

Dr. Richard Hobbs, the president of American Academy of Medical Acupuncture (AAMA), addressed that "Why is it so hard to connect the dots between concepts of Chinese medicine and Western science? " at the 21st annual AAMA symposium in Fort Worth, Texas (April 2009).

Capsi et al. (2000) proposed that studying the "ABC language" of the most common CAM disciplines in medical schools, along with the conventional curriculum, would help to educate a new generation of physicians with a better ability to communicate with CAM providers. Like trainees in many other professions, allopathic medical students are required to learn both the vocabulary (medical terms) and the grammar of almost all biomedical disciplines. Indeed, going through medical school is very much about learning this new biomedical jargon. If we are taught only 1 set of vocabulary, communication is less rich and therefore at times less effective, and if we miss words, we often miss concepts (Caspi et al., 2000).

However, the concept of TCM was established more than 3,000 years ago, and the ancient "physicians" and "scientists" in China used their own feelings and terminology to analyze health and illness. Do we need to educate and explain to CWM students and physicians the concepts of *Qi*, meridians, and *Yin*/*Yang*? A better solution is to translate the ancient words and concepts used in CAM to modern CWM terminology. Of course, this should only be done if the concepts of TCM are scientifically supported.

According to TCM, "Acupuncture is believed to restore the balance of *Yin* and *Yang.*" This can be translated into the CWM terminology as "Acupuncture restores the balance between the parasympathetic and sympathetic systems" (Takahashi, 2011) (Figure 1.2).

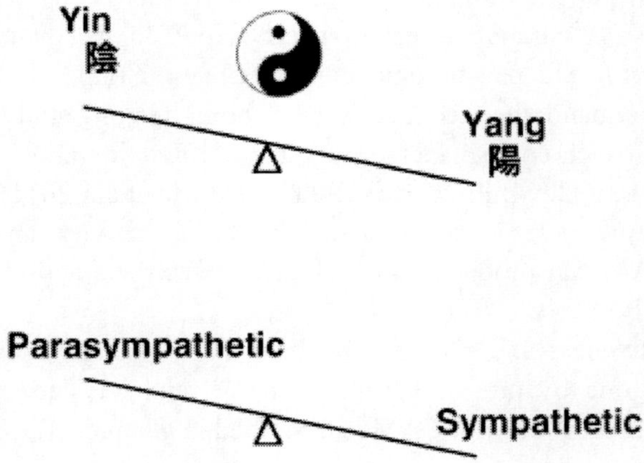

Figure 1.2. Translation from TCM (upper panel) to CWM (lower panel).

The medical training of CAM is basically possible, once we have succeeded in creating a common language. In the last decade, the mechanisms of various CAM procedures have widely been studied using our modern techniques of anatomy, physiology, biochemistry, pharmacology and molecular biology (see Chapter III and IV). Now, we are ready to build a concrete bridge between CAM practitioners and CWM physicians.

2.2. Poor Evidence of Efficacy and Mechanism

CAM methods are increasingly used by patients in the Western world to treat various diseases. Patients use these methodologies of their own accord, frequently against the advice of their physicians. More and more research is being conducted to convert the secrets behind the thousands of years of CAM experience.

It has been criticized that CAM promotes unscientific ideas and therapies. This puts us in conflict with evidence-based medicine. To test the efficacy of CAM, many randomized placebo-controlled clinical trials have been performed. However, the placebo arm sometimes produces equally effective results as the treatment arm. Therefore, Chang (2012) raised the following questions.

"How can we explain this? Is it logical to assume that since there is no scientific evidence for the efficacy of CAM, it is really the "placebo effect" that relieves the patient's ailment? Does the compassion a physician shows for his patient have a curative effect in itself? How do we distinguish a true biological effect from a psychological one? "(Chang, 2012).

On the other hand, the recent advance of brain imaging study suggests that emotional and psychological factors regulate the function and network in the brain (Wager et al., 2004; Price et al., 2007; Petrovic et al., 2011). It should be noted that CAM is able to regulate the brain activity and mind-body interaction. CAM can produce real biological effects via acting on our mind (psychologically).

The effectiveness and possible mechanism of various CAM procedures are described, one by one, in Chapter III, IV, and V. The mechanism of placebo effect associated with CAM is described in Chapter III.

3. Current Problems of CWM

Despite its great advance and establishment for the treatment of various diseases, there are several serious problems of CWM.

3.1. Less Attention to Self-Healing

It should be noted that our body has the ability to repair by themselves. Unfortunately, the concept of self-healing is absent in the education and practice of CWM. Most patients today have no confidence that their own body has an ability to heal by themselves. They think that they require medicine and treatment provided by the health care professionals.

3.2. Less Attention to a Whole Person

Human beings are more than just their physical bodies. Human beings have minds and emotions. CWM physicians only pay attention to the physical body. It is possible to treat physical disease through the mind and emotions. Future medicine should pay more attention on mind-body therapies.

3.3. Less Attention to Social Connectedness

Our survival depends on the ability to build mutually beneficial relationships with others. It is important for us to feel connected, to be trusted and loved. Feeling connected to others increases psychological and physical well-being (Brown et al., 2003; DeVries et al., 2003) and decreases the risk of depression and physical ailments (Hawkley et al., 2006). A sense of connectedness also increases empathetic responding as well as acts of trust and cooperation.

Despite the clear benefits of social connectedness, our society is becoming increasingly isolated and distrustful. Economical and social changes developed smaller social networks. It is crucial to pay attention to improve social connectedness of individuals, in order to decrease the risk of depression and physical ailments.

3.4. Less Attention to Preventive Medicine

Most of the chronic diseases in our population are diseases associated with our life style. Most of the diseases that we are managing are preventable diseases. They are frequently associated with our poor life style (diets, physical exercise, and social activities, etc.). In general, it is easier to prevent diseases than to manage them.

3.5. Less Attention to Doctor-Patient Relationship

The relationship between the practitioner and the patient is very important to the healing process. The relationship between the doctor and patient is the source of most of the emotional reward of practicing medicine. However, the time that doctors spend with the patients has become very short. Many doctors today only have 5-10 minutes to spend with the patient. When the system makes this so short, much of the satisfaction of practicing medicine disappears.

3.6. Adverse Effects of Drugs

Adverse effects are particularly important in pharmacology. Adverse effects, like therapeutic effects of drugs, are a function of dosage or drug levels at the target organs. Adverse effects can be reduced by careful and precise pharmacokinetics. Adverse effects may also be caused by drug interactions. This often occurs when patients fail to inform their physician and pharmacist of all the medications they are taking, including herbal and dietary supplements. Drug-drug and food-drug interactions may also occur.

In general, most drugs have a large list of non-severe or mild adverse effects which do not rule out continued usage. These effects, which have a widely variable incidence according to individual sensitivity, include nausea, dizziness, diarrhea, malaise, vomiting, headache, dermatitis, dry mouth, etc. These can be considered as forms of pseudo-allergic reactions, as not all users experience these effects.

3.7. Intoxication with Capitalism

Capitalism is an economic system that is based on private ownership of the means of production and the creation of goods or services for profit. Capitalism also includes competitive markets, wage labor and capital accumulation. For capitalism to function, the consumer must have control of spending and enough information to be a wise shopper in his/her own self-interest. In the US healthcare, the consumer/patient has virtually no control over who will provide service or what service will be provided. If the consumer/patient does not pay for what he/she is consuming under these conditions, how can any patient be the rational consumer on which capitalism depends? (Medical-Malprocess, 2010). It seems likely that the health care system suffers from being too intoxicated with capitalism.

3.7.1. High Profits of Pharmaceutical Companies

The pharmaceutical companies enjoy higher profits than any other industry. In 2002, the top 10 pharmaceutical companies in the US had a median profit margin of 17%, compared with only 3% for all the other industries on the Fortune 500 list. Subtracting losses from gains, those 10 companies made more in profits that year than the other 490 companies put together. Pfizer, the world's No. 1 pharmaceutical company, had a profit margin of 26% of sales in 2002. Its hefty cash flow was largely due to a line up of blockbuster drugs, including the cholesterol medication (Lipitor), anti-depressant (Zoloft) and allergic medicine (Zyrtec) (Pattison et al., 2003).

Of the top 10 pharmaceutical companies in the world, 5 are European and 5 are American, but all of them have US as their major profit center. In the US, many un-insured patients are charged more for drugs than those who have large insurance companies to bargain for them. Moreover, the prices of top selling drugs are routinely jacked up in the US at 2 to 3 times the general rate of inflation (Pattison et al., 2003).

The purpose of the pharmaceutical industry is to increase sales of drugs for ongoing diseases and to find new diseases to market existing drugs. In 2003, Aaron et al. reported that the pharmaceutical industry has the largest lobby in Washington, DC. There are more pharmaceutical lobbyists than members of the congress and it gives copiously to political campaigns (Aaron et al., 2003).

Advertising also expands the total market. Pharmaceutical companies increasingly promote diseases to fit drugs, rather than the reverse. They try to persuade wealthy people who are suffering from conditions that need long-term treatment. Thus, many normal people come to believe that they have dubious or exaggerated ailments such as generalized anxiety disorder, erectile dysfunction, and premenstrual dysphoric disorder etc. (Angell, 2004).

The high prescription drug expenditures lead to the struggle with rising health costs. Although outpatient prescriptions accounted for only 12% of US personal health care expenditures in 2002, they were its fastest growing component, increasing at an unsustainable rate of about 15% per year (Levit et al., 2004).

3.7.2 Financial Ties between Medical Professionals and Pharmaceutical Companies

It is generally accepted that prices should be high to cover their research and development costs for the big pharmaceutical companies. However, it seems that prices are high to cover their marketing costs. The big pharmaceutical companies have spent more on marketing and administration than on anything else. Throughout the 1990s, the top 10 companies in the world consistently spent about 35% of sales on marketing and administration, and only 11-14% on research and development (The-Henry-J-Kaiser-Family-Foundation, 2001). Among the top 10 US companies in 2002, expenditures for marketing and administration were 31% of sales, compared with only 14% for research and development. That comes to $67 billion dollars of their $217 billion in sales (Pattison et al., 2003).

Marketing includes expenditures for education of medical professionals. The medical profession has largely abdicated its responsibility to educate medical students and doctors in the use of prescription drugs. Pharmaceutical companies now support most continuing medical education, medical conferences and meetings of professional associations (Relman, 2001). In addition, the pharmaceutical industry is an extremely important source of funding for continuing medical education: 35% of the estimated $9–$14 billion that industry spends each year on pharmaceutical marketing goes toward educational support (Campbell et al., 2007).

The financial ties between doctors and pharmaceutical companies have come under intense scrutiny in recent years. Angell (2009) argues that the mission of doctors is fundamentally different to the mission of pharmaceutical companies and that the ties between them should be completely cut. She insisted that pharmaceutical companies are investor owned businesses with a responsibility to maximize profits for their shareholders. That is quite different from the mission of the medical profession, which is to provide the best care possible for patients (Angell, 2009).

3.7.3. Financial Incentives of Doctors

Once doctors own hospitals or test equipment, they tend to order unnecessary and expensive tests and procedures in order to make money. On the contrary, when they are paid a fixed sum of money, they tend to defer doing medical activities/cares. Thus, financial incentives could encourage doctors to behave in ways that are counter to the patients' welfare (Medical-Malprocess, 2010).

3.7.4. Insurance Industry

Private insurers maximize profits by spending as little as possible of their collected premiums. Government insurers also seek to spend as little as possible in order to stay within budget. The medical insurance industry suffers from the contradictory incentives built into our current healthcare system. Patients want their insurers to pay for whatever medical care they need or want. Shareholders want insurers to pay out as little as they can in order to maximize profits. Taxpayers want government insurers to pay out as little as possible to avoid tax increases. Incentives discourage providing care (Medical-Malprocess, 2010).

3.8. Expensive Medical Cost

There are two main reasons that health care costs are too expensive. (1) CWM does not practice to prevent disease, forcing practitioners to manage existing diseases. (2) The treatments that we depend on are high-tech treatments. Medical students and doctors of CWM don't currently have the opportunities to learn the beneficial effects and mechanisms of low-tech procedures, such as meditation, manual therapy, and exercise (Weil, 2011).

Insurance companies are willing to pay for drugs, expensive diagnostic tests, surgery, and high-tech inventions, but pay little attention to effective low-tech methods. Insurance will not pay doctors to consult with patients on how to improve their diet, how to reduce stress, or how to maintain daily exercise. The bills are coming from the pharmaceutical industry, manufacturers of medical equipment, and the insurance industry. All are making a lot of money from the present medical care system (Weil, 2011).

SUMMARY

Although interest in CAM has increased dramatically over the past decade, the efficacy of CAM needs to be proven by our current medical knowledge and technology. There is a huge gap between CWM and CAM, mainly due to the lack of a common language and common concepts.

CWM pays less attention to the importance of self-healing, whole person methodologies, preventive medicine, doctor-patient relationships, and social connectedness. CWM is also too intoxicated with capitalism. As the mechanisms of various CAM procedures have been widely studied through modern Western techniques, it's time to build a concrete bridge between CAM and CWM.

Chapter 2

Concept of Integrative Medicine

Integrative medicine combines mainstream medical therapies (CWM) and certain CAM therapies for which there is some high-quality scientific evidence of safety and effectiveness. Integrative medicine can cover the current problems of CWM by integrating the efficacy of both CWM and CAM.

1. Self-Healing

According to Dr. Weil, the director of Arizona Center of Integrative medicine, integrative medicine is a healing oriented medicine (Weil, 2011). Integrative medicine emphasizes the innate healing mechanism of the human body. Our bodies have the ability to diagnose problems themselves, to repair them, to regenerate, and to get back into the balance of health. The very important philosophical difference of integrative medicine from CWM is the emphasis on the human body's capacity for self-healing (Weil, 2011).

It should be noted that emotional impact, expectation, intension, or conditioning sometimes can alter the brain activity and its networking (See Chapter III), resulting in the stimulation of various neurotransmitters and neuropeptides, which lead to the beneficial effects for well-being. CWM has developed different kinds of agonists to treat diseases and symptoms, but CWM should focus more on how to activate/upregulate the endogenous substances, rather than the exogenous administration of drugs. The development of the procedure that activates endogenous substances, which may promote the process of self-healing, is one of the most important developments for the future of medicine.

By stimulating the mind-body connection through active procedures like meditation, Yoga, Tai-chi, Qi-gong, and auto-suggestions, we could upregulate/activate endogenous substances by ourselves. Through passive procedures like manual therapies, hypnosis, and doctor-patient relationships, we could also upregulate/activate endogenous substances in order to promote self-healing.

Placebo effect is a simple example of self-healing. Almost all the doctors dislike the placebo effects, because they think that placebo effects are non-specific and/or psychological. However, recent brain imaging studies demonstrated that highly active neuronal processes are mediated by psychological mechanisms such as expectation and conditioning and that brain networks and signaling systems are involved in the placebo response (Lieberman et al., 2004; Zubieta et al., 2009) (See Chapter III).

2. Human Beings

Human beings are more than just their physical bodies. Human beings have minds and emotions. It is possible to treat physical diseases through the mind and emotions. There is a great deal of evidence that mind-body therapies (meditation, hypnosis, Yoga, Tai-chi, Qi-gong, and music therapy) are beneficial for physical diseases. It is also possible to treat mental diseases through the physical approach. There is evidence that manual therapies (acupuncture and massage) are effective for mental diseases. The beneficial effects and mechanism of mind-body therapies and manual therapies are described in Chapter III and IV, respectively.

3. Preventive Medicine

Prevention can be categorized into three components. (1) Health promotion activities to prevent the actual occurrence of a specific illness or disease. (2) Health maintenance activities for early detection or screening and treatment of disease and limitation of disability. (3) Recovery or rehabilitation of a disease or condition after the disease has developed (Golbidi et al., 2012). Future medicine should pay great attention to all aspects of a person's life style, including diets, daily physical activities, rest, sleep, hobby, social interaction, etc. This focus gives us great power to practice effective preventive medicine.

4. Doctor-Patient Relationship

The relationship between the practitioner and the patient is important to the healing process. It is often said that CWM treats the diagnosis, whereas TCM treats the person. It has been demonstrated that the features of clinician-patient communication can predict health outcomes after the consultation. Street et al. (2009) emphasized that clinicians and patients can maximize the therapeutic effects of communication by explicitly orienting communication to achieve intermediate outcomes, such as trust, mutual understanding, adherence, social support, self-efficacy associated with improved health (Street et al., 2009).

As described in Chapter III, placebo effects are highly dependent on the practitioner-patient relationship. Through the positive and strong psychological interaction with the practitioner, oxytocin (OXT) neuron is activated in the patient's brain, which mediates the improvement of patients' health (See Chapter IV and VII).

5. Social Connectedness

Social activity is related to beneficial effects on the cardiovascular, endocrine, and immune systems. Social connectedness may have stress-buffering effects (Uchino et al., 1996). It is important for us to feel connected, to be trusted and loved. Feeling connected to others increases psychological and physical well-being and decreases the risk of depression and physical ailments.

Social interactions have a profound effect on health. People with a higher quality of social relationships show a lower risk of death (Seeman, 1996), while social isolation has been shown as a major risk factor for mortality (House et al., 1988). The most important protective factors among men were married status and frequent contacts with close friends and relatives (Berkman et al., 1979). Social activities may have modifying effects on life stresses and risk factors associated with mortality (Welin et al., 1985). Social activities and psychological coping styles reduce the deleterious effects of stress and thus reduce the risk of disease in a non-specific way (Cassel, 1976). Unfortunately, our society is becoming increasingly isolated and distrustful. It seems that technological, economical, and social changes have developed less trustworthiness among us.

Buddhist traditions have emphasized the importance of cultivating connection and love toward others through techniques such as loving-kindness meditation (LKM). This practice, in which one directs compassion and wishes for well-being toward real or imagined others, is designed to create changes in emotion and motivation (Salzberg, 1995). Surprisingly, the practice of LKM decreased chronic low back pain, psychological distress, and anger (Carson et al., 2005). Thus, it is highly conceivable that giving compassion and empathy to others is beneficial for the givers. It has been shown that providing social support is more beneficial than receiving it to reduce mortality in humans (Brown et al., 2003). Numerous studies reveal protective effects of volunteering on mental and physical health (Piliavin et al., 2007).

A positive social interaction is bidirectional, involving both giving and receiving empathy/care. It has been shown that giving affection and empathy to others is a key factor in upregulating hypothalamic OXT expression (Babygirija et al., 2012a). As OXT is linked to health-promoting cardiovascular, metabolic, analgesic, anti-inflammatory, and anti-stress effects, upregulated OXT expression would help to maintain our mental and physical health (see Chapter VII). It is important to reconsider Buddhist traditions of cultivating connection and compassion toward others in order to maintain our well-being.

> "If you want others to be happy, practice compassion. If you want to be happy, practice compassion." (Dalai Lama).

6. Integration of CWM and CAM

At present, it remains unclear (1) whether a true integration of CAM and CWM is even possible, (2) what this integration would look like, and (3) whether we are ready for the new era of medicine that would then result (Caspi et al., 2000).

Some CAM therapies are passive (acupuncture, massage, music therapy, hypnosis), while others require active patient participation (Yoga, Tai-chi, Qi-gong, meditation) (Deng et al., 2005). Patient preference is an important issue, as many patients prefer passive interventions, while others seek active means of participating in their own care. Still other patients prefer both, depending on the problem they hope to address. It is highly recommended that patients participate in active procedures to improve well-being and promote self-healing. Primary care providers can play a vital role in encouraging their patients to participate in these practices. Clinicians have the opportunity to educate their patients on the health benefits of these exercises and refer them to local centers where classes are offered. As a low-cost and low-impact exercise, a prescription for these serves as an effective alternative for individuals in need of an exercise program.

Collaboration of CWM and CAM should be developed for future medicine. We can change the situation through the education of doctors and medical students. We need to educate the public, to teach people how to take greater responsibility for their health. We also need to demonstrate that integrative medicine works better and cost-less than CWM for the management of common diseases.

SUMMARY

Both CWM and CAM approaches should truly be integrated into a holistic concept. For integrative medicine, self-healing, whole person (body, mind, and spirit), and social connectedness are taken into account, including all aspects of an individual's lifestyle. Integrative medicine also emphasizes the therapeutic relationship between the patients and their physicians.

Chapter 3

MIND-BODY MEDICINE

Cooperation between the body and the mind is emphasized in facilitating and achieving well-being. Changes in the body influence and facilitate emotional and cognitive processing. Mind–body interventions, combined use of body and mind training, covers a variety of techniques to enhance the mind's capacity to affect bodily functions and symptoms. These techniques include meditation, Yoga, Tai-chi, Qi-gong, hypnosis, autogenic training, etc.

1. MEDITATION

Meditation is a practice of mental silence, in which the activity of the mind is minimized without reducing the level of alertness. The foundation of meditation practice is rooted in the principles of self-observation of immediate psychic activity, training one's level of awareness, and cultivating an attitude of acceptance of process rather than content (Ospina et al., 2007; Ospina et al., 2008).

Meditation can be defined to include any of a family of practices in which the practitioner trains an individual to consciously calm his/her mind in order to realize some benefit or achieve inner peace or harmony. Despite lack of consensus in the scientific literature on a definition of meditation, most researchers agree that meditation implies a form of mental training that requires either stilling or emptying the mind (Chen et al., 2012a).

Although pharmacological approaches and more traditional forms of psychotherapy have strong empirical support for reducing anxiety, many patients are turning to meditation as an alternative approach to reduce stress and anxiety. Meditation offers a therapeutic and often spiritual approach that avoids side effects of medications. The potential regulatory functions of meditation practices on attention and emotion processes have a long-term impact on the brain and behavior.

Meditation is a whole package of mind–body exercise with possibility of change in life style or attitude, which includes both specific and non-specific effects. Although people with anxiety symptoms can find meaningful benefits through the meditation, it is not clear whether these benefits are mediated through placebo, expectation, or self-suggestion. The potential mechanism of placebo effects is described later in this Chapter.

Originally, meditation is a spiritual practice in many religions. Nowadays, it can be practiced by anyone regardless of his/her religions to facilitate a greater sense of calmness or awareness. There are several meditation techniques, such as mantra meditation, Zen meditation, and loving-kindness meditation (LKM) (Phongsuphap et al., 2008). Mantra meditation is associated with Hinduism in India, while Zen meditation and LKM are associated with Buddhism in Japan and Tibet, respectively (Figure 3.1).

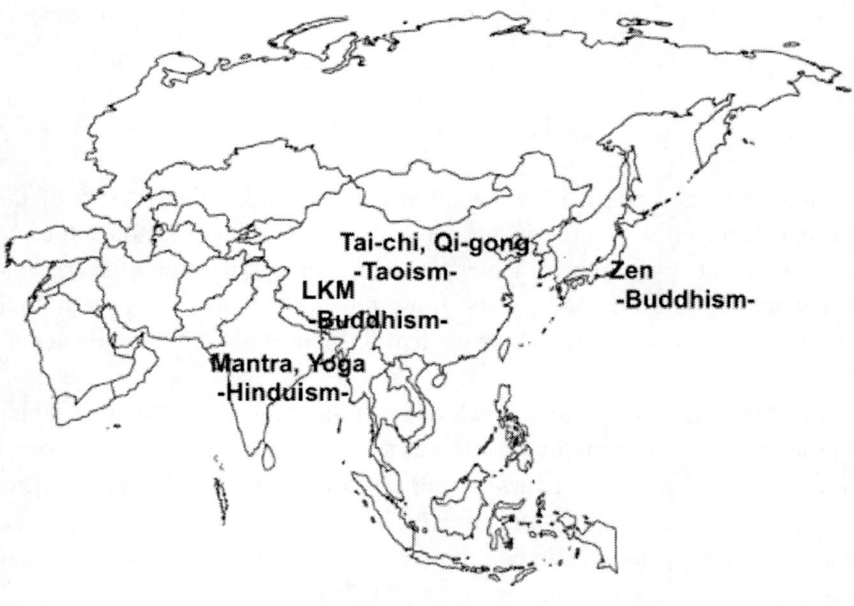

Figure 3.1. Different types of meditation-related techniques in the world.

1.1. Two Styles of Meditation

Among various practices of meditation, there are two styles that are commonly studied, focused attention (FA) meditation and open monitoring (OM) meditation.

FA is associated with maintaining focus on a specific object, often the changing sensation or flow of the breath or an external object (Lutz et al., 2008). When attention drifts from the object of focus to a distracting sensory, cognitive or emotional event, the practitioner is taught to acknowledge the event and to disengage from it by gently returning the attention back to the object of meditation. FA practitioner likely engages in cognitive reappraisal by repeatedly reinterpreting distracting events.

In contrast, OM is associated with a non-directed acknowledgement of any sensory, emotional or cognitive event that arises in the mind (Lutz et al., 2008). While practicing OM, the practitioner experiences the current sensory or cognitive event without evaluation, interpretation, or preference. OM practice is associated with a non-evaluative and non-elaborative mental stance. OM involves a complete lack of higher order appraisal (Zeidan et al., 2012).

FA and OM are usually combined, whether within a single session or over the course of a practitioner's training. These styles are found with some variation in several meditation traditions, including Zen meditation and Tibetan Buddhism (Lutz et al., 2008). In traditional Buddhist practice, novice meditators are first instructed to concentrate on observing the breath. Over time, as a meditator's ability to sustain attention on breath increases, he/she is gradually instructed to broaden his/her attention to other external and internal stimuli.

1.2. Mindfulness

Mindfulness is a state of mind that can be experienced during meditation. Mindfulness has been described as a practice of learning to focus attention on moment-by-moment experience with an attitude of curiosity, openness and acceptance (Marchand, 2012).

Several definitions of mindfulness have been used in modern psychology. According to various prominent psychological definitions, mindfulness refers to a psychological quality that involves bringing one's complete attention to the present experience or involves paying attention in a particular way. Practicing mindfulness can help people to begin to recognize their habitual patterns of mind, which have developed out of awareness over time and this allows practitioners to respond in new rather than habitual ways to their life (Shapiro et al., 2006; Carmody et al., 2009).

According to the teachings of the Buddha, mindfulness is an attentive awareness of the reality of things. The Buddha advocated that one should establish mindfulness in one's day-to-day life maintaining a calm awareness of one's bodily functions, sensations, objects of consciousness, and consciousness itself. Mindfulness practice, inherited from the Buddhist tradition, is being employed in Western psychology to alleviate a variety of mental and physical conditions including, anxiety, and depression (Shapiro et al., 2006; Carmody et al., 2009).

Mindfulness related health benefits are associated with enhancements in cognitive control, emotion regulation, positive mood, and acceptance (Grossman et al., 2004). Moreover, meditation has been shown to reduce cortisol and catecholamine level that trigger anxiety and stress responses (Ospina et al., 2007; Ospina et al., 2008; Zeidan et al., 2012).

1.3. Zen Meditation

Zen meditation is one of the main Buddhist meditations belonging to the pole of mindfulness meditation (Figure 3.2). Zen meditation comprehends various types of practices whose difficulty levels usually grow with the meditators' experience. The practitioners count their breaths so as to focus their attention. With ongoing practice, counting is omitted and the meditators remain simply aware of the present experience. This practice is called "*Shikantaza* "or "simply sitting" and is considered the most advanced form of Zen meditation. Zen meditation was found to reduce stress and blood pressure, and be efficacious for a variety of conditions, as suggested by positive findings in therapists and musicians (Chiesa, 2009).

As mentioned above, FA meditation involves the voluntary focusing of attention on a chosen object, such as a subset of localized sensations caused by breathing. OM meditation involves non-reactive monitoring of the content of experience from moment to moment. Although both FA and OM practices are combined over the course of Zen meditation training, FA on breathing movements in the lower abdomen (*Tan-Tien*) is considered the fundamental technique that is commonly practiced by Zen monks, who breathe more slowly during meditation practice and spend more time breathing out than breathing in (Kubota et al., 2001). The focusing of attention on lower abdominal breathing is practiced particularly in the initial stages of Zen meditation training by monks. Indeed, stress reduction is associated with slow, deep, regular, and diaphragmatic-abdominal breathing (Chapell, 1994).

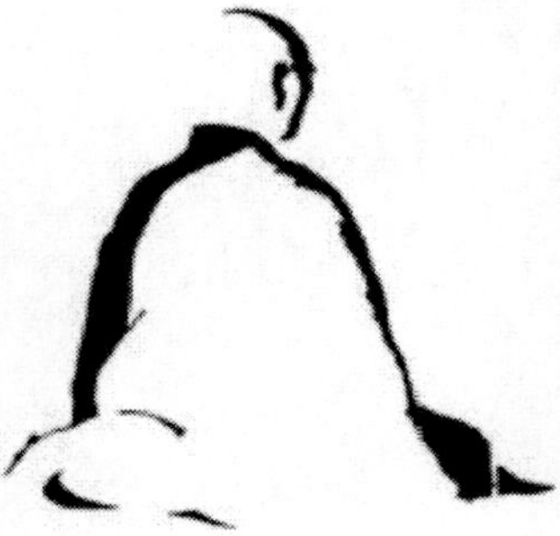

Figure 3.2. Zen meditation.

1.4. Loving-Kindness Meditation (LKM)

Compassion is the virtue of empathy for the suffering of others. It is regarded as the fundamental part of human love, and a cornerstone of greater social interconnection and humanism. The cultivation of loving-kindness is a popular form of meditation in Buddhism (Figure 3.3). LKM is a quiet, contemplative, mind-training practice used to cultivate positive emotions, such as friendliness, warmth, caring, joy, equanimity, and compassion. This practice begins with the meditator cultivating loving-kindness toward themselves, then their loved ones, friends, teachers, strangers, enemies, and finally toward all sentient beings. To cultivate positive emotions, various techniques are used to arouse feelings of loving-kindness (visualizing oneself or the person smiling or being joyous, reflecting on the positive qualities of the person, or using brief mental phrases) (Salzberg, 1995). Through this practice, feelings of anger, resentment, and anxiety can be released.

In the Tibetan Buddhist tradition, this practice is associated with "*tonglen*", whereby one breathes out (sends) happiness and breathes in (receives) suffering. Buddhist traditions have emphasized the importance of cultivating connection and love toward others through LKM. This practice is designed to create changes in emotion, motivation, and behavior in order to promote positive feelings and kindness toward oneself and others (Salzberg, 1995).

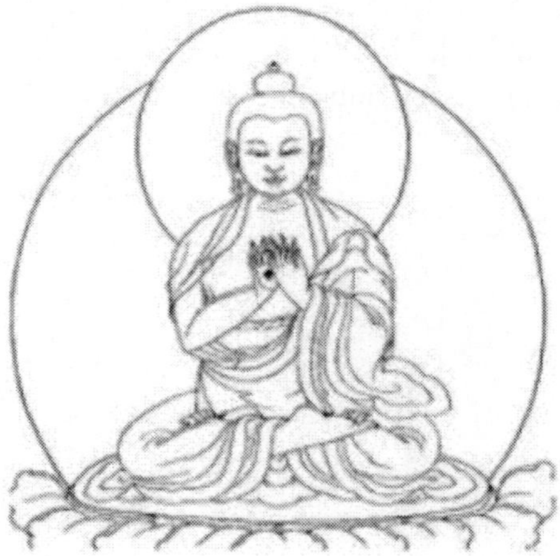

Figure 3.3. Buddhism.

Randomized clinical research has demonstrated that the practice of LKM has significant beneficial effects, such as decreased chronic low back pain, reduced psychological distress, reduced anger, and increased social connectedness (Carson et al., 2005; Hutcherson et al., 2008). There is also evidence that through the cultivation of positive emotions with LKM practice, individuals experience decreased illness symptoms as well as an increase in a broader range of personal resources such as social support, purpose in life, and increased mindfulness (Fredrickson et al., 2008), which predicted greater life satisfaction and reduced symptoms of depression.

1.5. Brain Activity during Meditation

Two neuroimaging techniques developed over the last 10-15 years, functional magnetic resonance imaging (fMRI) and positron emission tomography (PET) have excellent spatial resolution (Figure 3.4). The wealth of information these tools provide concerning specific brain regions has revolutionized neuroscience, allowing scientists to identify activity inside the brain during a wide variety of tasks. Following the growing interest in mindfulness techniques, a handful of studies using these tools to investigate meditation have been published. However, it should be noted that fMRI and PET do not provide any information as to different types of neuron firing.

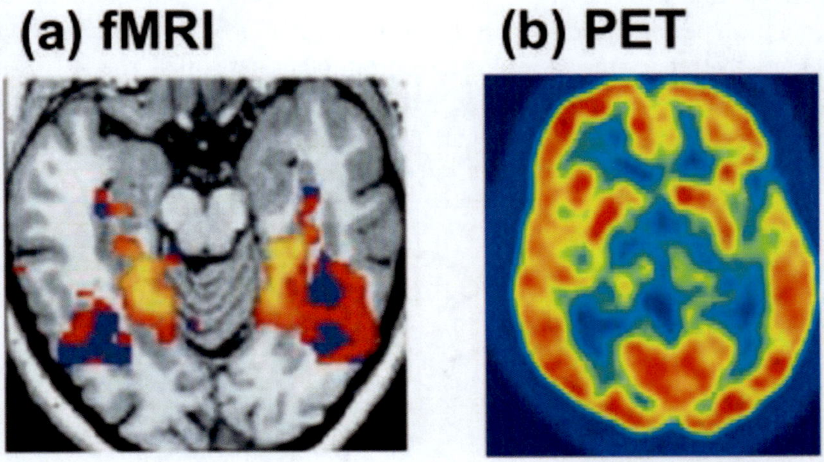

Figure 3.4. fMRI (left) and PET (right) image.

Meditation is associated with both state and trait-like effects. State effects refer to changes that occur in individuals while they actively meditate. In contrast, trait-like changes occur gradually over time as a consequence of sustained meditation practice and persist throughout the day. Trait-like effects are thought to result from stable, long-term transformations in brain activity and structure. With repetition, a mindfulness practice can create intentional states of brain activation that may ultimately become traits of the individual. New patterns of repeated neural circuit activation strengthen the synaptic connections and growth (neuro-plasticity).

A brain network including anterior cingulate cortex (ACC) and prefrontal cortex (PFC) has been shown to be an important mechanism for self-regulation of cognition and emotion (Allman et al., 2001) (Figure 3.5). The PFC is the anterior part of the frontal lobes of the brain, lying in front of the motor and premotor areas. This brain region is implicated in planning complex cognitive behavior, personality expression, decision-making and moderating social behavior. The basic activity of PFC is considered to be orchestration of thoughts and actions in accordance with internal goals.

The ACC is the frontal part of the cingulate cortex that resembles a collar form around the corpus callosum. It plays a role in a wide variety of autonomic functions (regulating blood pressure and heart rate) as well as rational cognitive functions (reward anticipation, decision-making, empathy and emotion). The sensitivity of the ACC to both reward and pain (Hampton et al., 2007) and evidence for ACC coupling to cognitive and emotional areas during task performance support the idea that the role of this brain region is to regulate the processing of information from other networks. The ACC serves as part of an executive attention network involved in the control of both cognition and emotion (Posner et al., 2007).

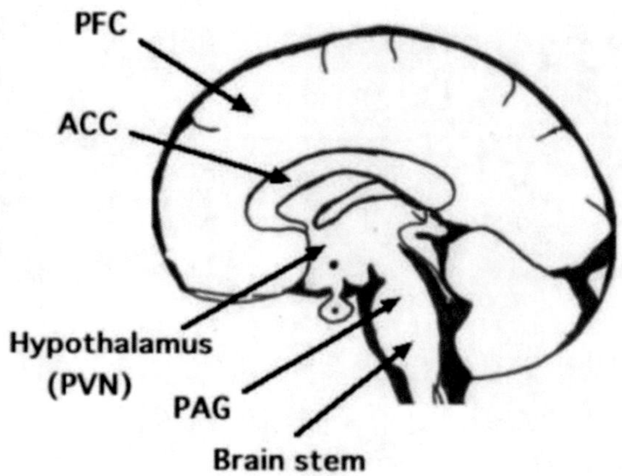

Figure 3.5. PFC and ACC in the brain.

The PFC is very sensitive to the detrimental effects of stress exposure. Prolonged stress exposure causes architectural changes in prefrontal dendrites (Cerqueira et al., 2008; Arnsten, 2009). The malfunctioning of PFC induced by stress is highly relevant to mental and physical health (Arnsten, 2009). It has been shown that the PFC and ACC were activated by various types of meditation, such as mindfulness meditation (Farb et al., 2007; Farb et al., 2012), Tibetan Buddhist meditation (Baron Short et al., 2007), Zen meditation (Yu et al., 2011), and Yoga meditation (Lazar et al., 2000; Froeliger et al., 2012). This suggests the possibility that meditation may re-organize the malfunction of PFC associated with stress.

To gain insight into the neurophysiological mechanisms involved in Zen meditation, Yu et al. (2011) evaluated the effects of FA on breathing movements in the lower abdomen in novices. The dynamic changes in the PFC were monitored by near-infrared spectroscopy during a 20-minute session of abdominal breathing in healthy volunteers. The level of oxygenated hemoglobin in the anterior PFC was significantly increased during FA on abdominal breathing, accompanied by a reduction in feelings of negative mood, compared to before the meditation session. Electroencephalography

(EEG) revealed the increased alpha band activity and decreased theta band activity during and after FA on abdominal breathing. EEG changes were correlated with a significant increase in whole blood serotonin (5-HT) levels. These results suggest that activation of the anterior PFC and 5-HT system may be responsible for the improvement of negative mood and EEG signal changes observed during FA on abdominal breathing (Yu et al., 2011).

Tang et al. (2009) adopted integrative mind body training (IBMT) from Tai-chi and Qi-gong and incorporated aspects of meditation and mindfulness training (Tang et al., 2009). Healthy volunteers were randomly assigned to an IBMT group or to a control group (relaxation training) for 5 days of short-term training (20 min per day). After 5 days of training, the IBMT group showed significantly greater improvement of performance in attention and positive mood, significantly reduced cortisol secretion following a stressful experience. Greater involvement of the autonomic nervous system was seen in the IBMT group during and after training. Brain imaging studies demonstrated stronger subgenual and adjacent ventral ACC activity in the IBMT group. These results indicated that IBMT improves regulation of the autonomic nervous system by a ventral mid frontal brain system (Tang et al., 2009).

After an 8 week-program of mindfulness practice, an increase in gray matter concentration within the left hippocampus was observed, compared to a waiting list control group. Whole brain analyses identified increases in the posterior cingulate cortex (PCC), and the cerebellum in the practice group, compared with the controls. These suggests that participation in mindfulness practice is associated with changes in gray matter concentration in brain regions involved in learning and memory processes, emotion regulation, self-referential processing, and perspective taking (Holzel et al., 2011).

Social anxiety disorder (SAD) is characterized by emotional and attentional biases as well as distorted negative self-beliefs. Previous studies showed exaggerated amygdala responses in SAD in response to social anxiety-related stimuli (Phan et al., 2006; Blair et al., 2008). Mindfulness-based stress reduction (MBSR) is an established program to reduce symptoms of stress, anxiety, and depression. After a 2 month training of MBSR, 14 patients of SAD were examined by fMRI. Compared with baseline, MBSR completers showed improvement in anxiety and depression symptoms and self-esteem. MBSR completers also showed reduced amygdala activity and increased activity in brain regions implicated in attentional deployment. MBSR-related reductions in social anxiety symptom severity were associated with increased MBSR-related neural responses in middle occipital brain regions implicated in visual attention (Goldin et al., 2010).

2. Yoga

Yoga means to yoke or to join together, coming from Sanskrit in Hindu astrology (Figure 3.1). A description of the physical Yoga postures was found in the Yoga Sutras, which was written in 3,000 BC by Patanjali, a Sanskrit scholar and an Indian physician. Yoga practice typically combines stretching exercises and different poses with meditation (Figure 3.6). Yoga is designed to stretch and tone the muscles and to keep the spine and joints flexible. Yoga poses are generally done with deep, diaphragmatic breathing that is thought to increase oxygen flow to the brain. A series of poses are performed slowly and sequentially, concentrating each movement on the deep abdominal breathing that accompanies each movement. Movements between poses are considered as important as maintaining a pose, and typically the poses are held for 4 or 5 breaths depending on the different teaching styles of Yoga. It has been suggested that the bending, twisting and stretching movements also massage the internal organs and glands.

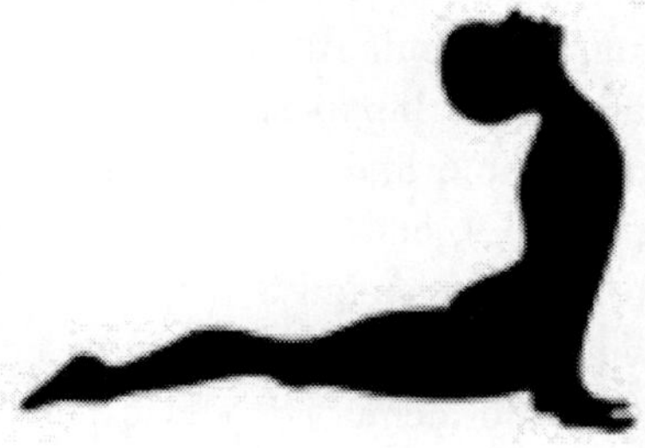

Figure 3.6. Yoga.

2.1. Psychological Effects

Yoga has been shown to have psychological effects: decreasing anxiety (Shelov et al., 2009) and increasing feelings of emotional, social, and spiritual well-being (Williams et al., 2005). Compared to waiting-list group, those who participated in the Yoga training (two weekly 90-min sessions) showed decreased stress, anxiety, fatigue and depression (Michalsen et al., 2005). Yoga reduced job stress of fire fighters in the fire stations (Cowen, 2010). Performance anxiety has also been decreased in professional musicians following Yoga (Khalsa et al., 2009). Two months of trial Yoga led to decreased depression (Uebelacker et al., 2010). The decreased depression induced by Yoga was associated with the changes in brain activity and decreased cortisol levels. Weekly Yoga sessions increased alpha waves (sign of increased relaxation) and decreased cortisol levels (Kamei et al., 2000)

Yoga also reduced sleep disturbances following 6 months of practice in a geriatric population. Yoga showed a significant decrease in the time taken to fall asleep, an increase in the total number of hours slept and in the feeling of being rested in the morning (Manjunath et al., 2005). Immediate effects of Yoga on anxiety following one session have also been noted (Telles et al., 2009).

The early breast cancer outpatients were randomly assigned to Yoga or brief supportive therapy prior to the surgery. The Yoga sessions lasted 60 min daily while the control group was given supportive therapy during their hospital visits as a part of routine care. Self reported state anxiety and trait anxiety were significantly decreased in Yoga group compared to the control group (Rao et al., 2009). In another study, women with metastatic breast cancer showed less pain and fatigue and increased relaxation after one year of weekly Yoga (Carson et al., 2007). In breast cancer patients, weekly Yoga sessions similarly led to improved quality of life and reduced anxiety (Speed-Andrews et al., 2010; Ulger et al., 2010).

2.2. Anti-Nociceptive Effects (Analgesic Effects)

Adults with chronic low back pain were randomly assigned to the Yoga, therapeutic exercise, or self-care group. After 12 weeks of Yoga sessions, back pain was significantly reduced and back-related function was superior in the Yoga group, compared to the therapeutic exercise and self-care group (Sherman et al., 2005; Williams et al., 2005). Yoga group showed decreased disability scores, compared to the control group. Yoga group also had greater increase in spinal flexion (Chattha et al., 2008; Tekur et al., 2008).

Individuals with migraine headaches were randomly assigned to the Yoga, or self-care group. After 3 months of weekly sessions, the intensity and frequency of headache ratings, the anxiety and depression scores and the medication use were lower in the Yoga group, compared to those of the self-care group (John et al., 2007).

Yoga has also been effective for osteoarthritis of the hands and knees. After 8-week Yoga sessions, the participants experienced less pain, and improved physical functions (Garfinkel et al., 1994; Kolasinski et al., 2005).

Once the patients with rheumatoid arthritis were given a biweekly Yoga program for 6 weeks, significant improvements were noted in pain and pain disability and related measures of depression, vitality and self-efficacy (Evans et al., 2010). Yoga participants after 12 weeks of weekly classes reported less pain killer use than the waiting list control group (Saper et al., 2009).

2.3. Cardiovascular Effects

Yoga typically leads to increased heart rate, but following prolonged training, exercise-induced heart rate increase will be decreased. When, the healthy participants were asked to step up and down the platform at a rate of 30 steps per minute for 5 min, heart rate and systolic blood pressure increased and diastolic blood pressure decreased. After two months of Yoga training, the exercise-induced increase in heart rate and systolic blood pressure were significantly reduced (Madanmohan et al., 2004).

The Yoga group practiced Yoga postures for 45 min daily for 3 months, while the control group performed flexibility exercises for 40 min and slow running for 20 min daily for 3 months. The men in the Yoga group showed a significant decrease in heart rate and blood pressure and greater aerobic performance, than the control group (Telles et al., 2000).

Yoga has been effective for the patients of hypertension (Cade et al., 2010). Following a daily Yoga practice (1 hr for 20 weeks), the participants had decreased blood pressure, blood glucose, cholesterol and triglycerides and improved subjective well-being and quality of life (Damodaran et al., 2002). Yoga is also beneficial for the patients with advanced coronary artery disease. Following one year of Yoga training, serum cholesterol level was reduced by 23% in the Yoga group, while the standard treatment control group showed a 4% reduction. The serum low density lipids was also significantly decreased in the Yoga group (26%), compared to the control group (3%) (Yogendra et al., 2004).

A dietary change plus Yoga group was compared with a group who only made dietary changes of coronary artery disease patients. After one year of weekly sessions, Yoga group had fewer anginal episodes, improved exercise capacity, decreased body weight and lower serum total cholesterol levels. Low-density lipoprotein (LDL)-cholesterol and triglyceride levels also decreased in Yoga group. Revascularization procedures (coronary angioplasty or bypass surgery) were less frequently required in Yoga group, and coronary angiography showed that more lesions regressed and fewer lesions progressed in the dietary change plus Yoga group (Manchanda et al., 2000). This suggests that multiple treatment procedures (dietary change plus Yoga) confounded the Yoga effects. Dietary and exercise changes may interact to develop complex effects.

2.4. Physical Effects

Yoga practice for 4 years resulted in a 3-pound lower weight gain among normal weight participants and a 19-pound lower weight gain among overweight participants (Kristal et al., 2005). Yoga for 12 weeks showed an overall reduction in food consumption, eating speed and food choices (McIver et al., 2009). A 6-day Yoga program led to decreased body mass index (BMI), waist and hip circumference, fat-free mass, total cholesterol, high-density lipoprotein and fasting serum leptin levels. Eating disorder symptoms have also decreased following Yoga (Telles et al., 2010). In healthy seniors, 3-6 months of weekly Yoga classes improved physical balance and flexibility (Oken et al., 2006; Schmid et al., 2010).

High school long distance runners were randomly assigned to participate in brief Yoga exercises, or a no intervention control condition. Participants assigned to Yoga exercises showed significant improvements in running performance relative to control condition participants. Yoga sessions in 8 weeks increased leg strength and leg muscle in healthy young adults (Hart et al., 2008).

2.5. Possible Mechanisms of Yoga

2.5.1. Attenuation of Stress Responses

Stress is a physical response to events that make us feel threatened or upset. When we sense danger, the body's defenses kick into high gear in a rapid, automatic process known as the "fight-or-flight" reaction, or the stress response. Stress affects the mind, body, and behavior in many ways, and everyone experiences stress differently. Stress stimulates corticotropin releasing factor (CRF) at the PVN, which promotes the release of adrenocorticotropin hormone (ACTH) from the anterior pituitary. Released ACTH stimulates the cortisol release from the adrenal grand. This pathway is called as hypothalamic-pituitary-adrenal (HPA) axis (Figure 3.7).

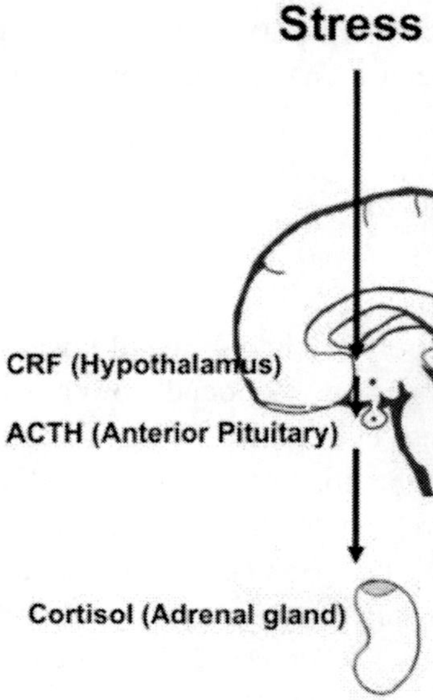

Figure 3.7. HPA axis in response to stress.

The sympathetic nervous system also gets triggered as a response to a physical or psychological stressor, leading to a cascade of physiological, behavioral, and psychological effects, primarily as a result of the released catecholamines. Over time, the constant state of hyper-vigilance resulting from repeated activation of the HPA axis and sympathetic nervous system can lead to dysregulation of the system and anxiety.

Yoga can improve physical and mental health through down-regulation of the HPA axis and the sympathetic nervous system. Studies showed that Yoga decreases levels of salivary cortisol (West et al., 2004; Michalsen et al., 2005) and urine catecholamine levels (Selvamurthy et al., 1998), resulting in reduced heart rate and systolic and diastolic blood pressure (Selvamurthy et al., 1998; Damodaran et al., 2002; Gokal et al., 2007).

West et al. (2004) compared the effects of Yoga to African dance, a vigorous form of exercise, and a college lecture. Both African dance and Yoga yielded significant improvements in perceived stress, with no significant changes noted in the lecture group. Dance intervention led to significant improvements in positive affect, while Yoga group remained unchanged and the lecture group experienced significant worsening. Both Yoga and dance group perceived their stress levels to be reduced. However, only Yoga group experienced significant reductions in levels of salivary cortisol. Levels of salivary cortisol significantly increased in the African dance group. These findings indicate that Yoga and exercise may both improve mood but affect the HPA axis differently (West et al., 2004).

By analyzing the electrocardiography (ECG), sympathetic and parasympathetic activity can be evaluated by heart rate variability (HRV) analysis non-invasively. The power in the high frequency (HF) band of HRV represents parasympathetic activities (Pomeranz et al., 1985). In contrast, the power in the low frequency (LF) band of HRV represents a combination of sympathetic and parasympathetic activities in humans (Pomeranz et al., 1985).

A significant reduction was noted in sympathetic nervous system activation in depressed patients following an 8-week Yoga intervention (Sarang et al., 2006; Shapiro et al., 2007). HRV study also showed that Yoga practice during the day appears to shift sympatho-vagal balance in favor of parasympathetic dominance during sleep on the following night (Patra et al., 2010). Thus, it is conceivable that Yoga exercises cause a shift toward parasympathetic nervous system dominance, possibly via direct vagal nerve stimulation (Innes et al., 2005).

Khattab et al. (2007) used a 24-hour ECG monitoring to compare Yoga practice versus park walking in Yoga practitioners. Yoga practitioners exhibited greater parasympathetic tone, during the Yoga intervention than during walking (Khattab et al., 2007).

Heart rates significantly decreased following a 6-week Yoga intervention, but not after aerobic cycling. No changes occurred in the parasympathetic tone following aerobic training, but increased in the parasympathetic tone in Yoga group (Bowman et al., 1997). This likely happens via stimulation of dermal and/or subdermal pressure receptors that are innervated by vagal afferent fibers, which ultimately project to the limbic system including hypothalamic structures involved in cortisol secretion (Field, 2011).

As described in Chapter IV, manual therapy (acupuncture and massage) stimulates vagal activity and decreases cortisol levels and depression. This is mediated via the somato-sensory stimulation of the skin and muscle. Effects of Yoga may be similar to those of manual therapy, because Yoga is a kind of self-massage from the rubbing of limbs against each other and against the floor. Manual therapy and Yoga both appear to stimulate pressure receptors under the skin, which in turn, leads to enhanced vagal activity and reduced cortisol. These physiological and biochemical changes would be expected to be accompanied by reduced depression and fewer pain syndromes and immune problems (Field, 2011).

2.5.2. Stimulation of Oxytocin (OXT) Release

Central oxytocin (OXT) plays an important role in mediating anti-stress effects, anti-nociceptive effects and social cognition (see Chapter VII). A recent study randomized schizophrenia patients to receive Yoga or remained waitlisted for 1 month. Consenting patients who participated, demonstrated significant benefits in emotional recognition following Yoga. However, no such benefit was demonstrated in waitlisted subjects. Blood samples were collected before and after Yoga or waitlist period. OXT levels rose significantly (nearly threefold) in Yoga group, but not in waitlisted group. This supports the possibility that OXT elevations are caused by Yoga. This mechanism may explain the benefits in social cognition as well as the well-being effect following Yoga (Bangalore et al., 2012).

As described above, the PFC and ACC were activated by Yoga (Lazar et al., 2000; Froeliger et al., 2012). It is conceivable to hypothesize that Yoga meditation activates PFC and ACC, which in turn stimulates hypothalamic OXT release. This results in reduced CRF expression and HPA axis activity (Figure 3.8).

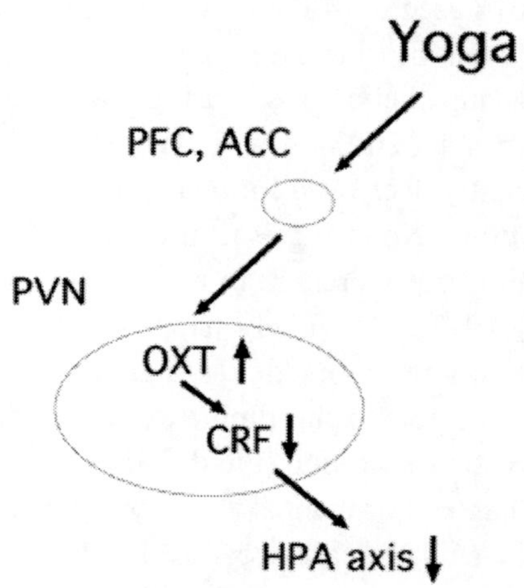

Figure 3.8. Yoga meditation may activate the PFC and ACC which in turn stimulates hypothalamic OXT release, resulting in reduced CRF expression and HPA axis activity.

3. TAI-CHI AND QI-GONG

Tai-chi and Qi-gong are closely associated with Taoism, Chinese philosophies and religions (Figure 3.1). The center doctrine of Taoism is focused on mind tranquility, and its goal is to achieve longevity by meditation and lifestyle modification. Although substantial variation within and between these practices exists, Tai-chi and Qi-gong are meditative exercises that coordinate gentle movements (Birdee et al., 2009) (Figure 3.9).

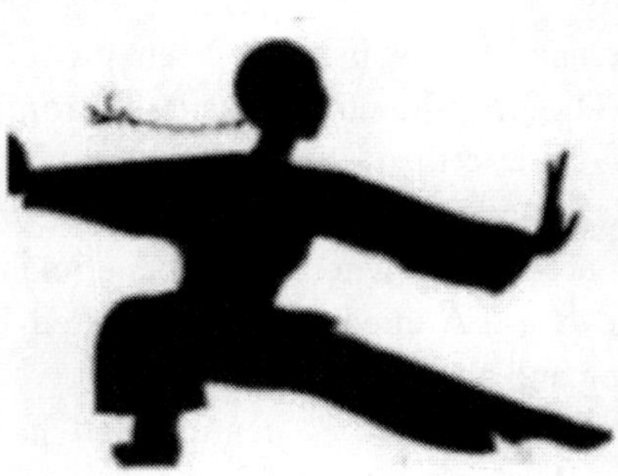

Figure 3.9. Tai-chi.

Tai-chi and Qi-gong are characterized by extreme slowness of movement, absolute continuity without break or pause, and a total focusing of awareness on the moment. Unlike most exercises that are characterized by muscular force and exertion, the movements of Tai-chi and Qi-gong are slow, gentle and light. The active concentration of the mind is instrumental in guiding the flow of the body's movements. Thus, Tai-chi and Qi-gong not only involves physical exercise, but also involves training of the mind, and this has prompted some to consider the practice of moving meditation. The main difference between Qi-gong and Tai-chi is that Tai-chi is a martial art form. Tai-chi movements can be faster to provide a form of self-defense, whereas this is not the case with the forms of Qi-gong.

From the perspective of TCM, all forms of meditation that are essentially mind-body integrative exercises are categorized as Tai-chi and Qi-Gong. These are defined as the skill of mind–body exercises that integrate body, breath, and mind adjustments into one, which addresses both psychological and physiological aspects of health (Allen et al., 2011).

As described in Chapter I, *Qi* in Chinese means vital energy, which is free flowing in the body along the energy channels called meridians. All Tai-chi and Qi-gong practices are based on the concept of *Qi*. Tai-chi and Qi-gong can be combined to facilitate energy cultivation and enhance training effects. Movements performed as part of Tai-chi and Qi-gong are used to aid *Qi* to flow smoothly, remove blockages, and increase general energy levels. Qi-gong uses deep, diaphragmatic breathing in conjunction with slow Tai-chi movements to bring our body, mind, and spirit into alignment and balance. The open and closed arm movements of Tai-chi are coordinated with breathing. Deep breathing in Qi-gong draws breath down into the "*Tan-Tien*" (the main energy center of the body), putting less pressure on lungs, and increasing lung capacity.

However, the presence of *Qi* has not been proved yet. The beneficial effects of Tai-chi and Qi-gong should be discussed from the viewpoint of our scientific knowledge. As described above, FA meditation is associated with maintaining focus on a specific object, such as flow of breath and an external object. Further studies are needed whether the beneficial effect of Tai-chi and Qi-gong are mediated via FA meditation associated with focus on deep diaphragmatic breathing and slow body movement.

Tai-chi was developed in the 17th century and had been practiced for centuries in China for health promotion, and it has gained popularity in Western societies. In the early 1990s, the number of papers about Tai-Chi published each year was less than 10, but now it exceeds 100 per year. Research papers on Tai-chi can be seen in the category of general medicine, sports medicine, rehabilitation, geriatrics, orthopedics and psychology.

Recent studies prove that Tai-chi is safe and effective for patients with cardiac, neurological and musculoskeletal disease. Tai-chi is beneficial for patients with coronary artery disease, heart failure, Parkinson's disease, stroke, traumatic brain injuries, arthritis, osteoporosis and chronic pain disorder (Komelski et al., 2012).

Tai-chi may be practiced in any environment without any special equipment. Classes are becoming increasingly prevalent in community and health care facilities. Allen and Meires (2011) proposed that Tai-chi therapy has the advantage of improving the physical and mental well-being for those with a variety of diseases and disorders (Allen et al., 2011).

3.1. Physical Effects

Qualitative information was gathered by Yau (2008) to gain an understanding of Tai-chi's meaning to those who practice it on a daily basis for 1 hour for an average of 8.5 years. Practicing Tai-chi clarifies life's significance and sense, and it gives way to a feeling of overall well-being and stamina. The participants placed a high importance on the social experience of group practice, which gave them a supportive network of friends who shared in their lives. The psychosocial and way-of-life aspects of Tai-chi practice led to better quality of life than the physical aspect. Tai-chi helped them have better memory, and better overall stress relief (Yau, 2008).

Cancer patients, particularly breast cancer patients, frequently experience debilitating side effects from the various modalities of treatment, including surgery, chemotherapy, and radiation therapy. Mustian et al. (2008) compared the effectiveness of Tai-chi vs psychosocial support for breast cancer survivors. Baseline measurements were obtained in the areas of aerobic capacity, muscular strength, flexibility, and quality of life. The interventional group received 12 weeks of Tai-chi classes, and the control group received psychosocial support, which emphasized coping skills and social interaction. Tai-chi group achieved significant improvements in aerobic capacity, handgrip strength, flexibility, and quality of life, with greater improvements achieved over time. The psychosocial support group revealed increases in only abduction under the flexibility measurements (Mustian et al., 2008).

Breast cancer survivors were randomly assigned to Tai-chi exercise or standard support therapy for 12 weeks (3 times/week for 60 min/session). Tai-chi group improved the total health-related quality of life, physical functioning, physical role limitations, social functioning, and general mental health. Plasma cortisol changes were associated with changes in physical role limitations and health perceptions (Sprod et al., 2012).

3.2. Anti-Stress Effects

Sleep disturbances are suffered by approximately 70% of those diagnosed with posttraumatic stress disorder (PTSD) (Ohayon et al., 2000). Slater and Hunt (1997) reported a decrease in nightmares after Tai-Chi exercise, as compared to a stretching exercise control group (Slater et al., 1997). In a randomized clinical trial with older adults, a 6-month Tai-chi program improved moderate sleep complaints. Thus, Tai-chi appears to be effective as a non-pharmacological approach to sleep enhancement for sleep-disturbed elderly individuals (Li et al., 2004). Incorporating Qi-gong and Tai-chi into the treatment may support the potential efficacy for survivors of torture and refugee trauma (Grodin et al., 2008).

3.3. Cardiovascular Effects

Tai-chi specifically has been offered as the ideal exercise for chronic heart failure patients (Yeh et al., 2008). Yeh et al. (2008) investigated Tai-chi's effectiveness in improving exercise capacity (Yeh et al., 2008). Tai-chi group received 1-hour classes twice per week for duration of 12 weeks. Exercise capacity, measured by a 6-minute walk test, significantly improved in Tai-chi participants. The patients in the Tai-chi classes reported a high level of satisfaction in participating in the therapy, and nearly all the patients intended to continue engaging in Tai-chi after completion of the study (Yeh et al., 2008).

3.4. Possible Mechanisms of Tai-Chi And Qi-Gong

3.4.1. Attenuation of HPA Axis

Tai-chi and Qi-gong are a slow and graceful form of exercise and meditation. Exercise has been shown to positively influence quality of life for those with a wide variety of medical illnesses, including multiple forms of cancer, hypertension, and chronic pain (Lee et al., 2007; Taylor-Piliae et al., 2007).

Tai-Chi has been shown to acutely decrease sympathetic nervous system activity, as measured by cardiac pre-ejection period (Motivala et al., 2006). Tai-chi has been shown to reduce cortisol levels, possibly implicating the HPA axis in Tai-chi-induced stress and anxiety reduction (Lee et al., 2004).

3.4.2. Stimulation of Parasympathetic Activity

After Tai-chi practice, parasympathetic tone was increased, while sympathetic tone decreased. Heart rate, systolic blood pressure, and diastolic blood pressure also decreased sequentially after Tai-chi. These suggest that Tai-chi enhance the vagal modulation and tilt the sympatho-vagal balance (Lu et al., 2003).

4. Placebo Effects

Prospective, double blind, placebo-controlled studies examining clinical problems are considered as gold standard for evidence-based medicine (EBM).

The term 'placebo' has its origin in the Latin '*placeo, placere*', meaning 'to please'. In general, the placebo effect is understood as an improvement in the symptoms and/or physiological functions of the organism as a reaction to non-specific and apparently inert factors, such as visual or verbal suggestion, taking pills, and fictitious surgery. Placebo effects are most commonly attributed to the symbolism exerted by the treatment on the positive expectations of the patient.

In modern medicine, the placebo effect has often been regarded as a nuisance particularly in clinical research. In general, most doctors dislike the placebo effects, because they think that placebo effects are non-specific and/or psychological. While the placebo responses in various medical conditions have been shown to follow few basic principles, the underlying neurobiology and the mediating hormonal and neuronal modulating processing have remained obscure (Enck et al., 2008). The placebo effect stem from highly active processes in the brain that are mediated by psychological mechanisms such as expectation and conditioning. Brain networks and signaling systems may be involved in the placebo response (Lieberman et al., 2004; Zubieta et al., 2009).

4.1. Placebo-Induced Analgesia

Opioid neurons play an important role to reduce painful sensation. Nociceptive messages from the spinal cord to the brain are suppressed by the descending inhibition system. Opioid neurons at the periaqueductal grey (PAG) play an important role of descending inhibition on the pain pathways (Millan, 2002) (Figure III-10).

It is widely accepted that placebo analgesia is partly mediated by the endogenous opioid system since the opioid receptor antagonist (naloxone) attenuates the placebo effect (Benedetti, 1996; Amanzio et al., 1999; Sauro et al., 2005). Among the modulating mechanisms of placebo analgesia, it is postulated that the expectation of lessening of pain stimulates production of endogenous opioids (Teixeira et al., 2010). However, there are differences between the two treatments. While opioids have direct pharmacological effects, acting on the descending pain inhibitory system, placebo analgesia depends on neocortical top-down mechanisms (Petrovic et al., 2011).

The PFC in the brain is responsible for executive function, which relates to abilities to differentiate among conflicting thoughts, determine good and bad, same and different, future consequences of current activities, working toward a defined goal, prediction of outcomes, expectation based on actions, etc.

Placebo analgesia is typically preceded by greater activation of the PFC during anticipation of pain, an effect that predicts reductions in pain perception and activity in pain-related brain regions (Petrovic et al., 2011). It has been suggested that the dorsolateral PFC has a primary role in maintaining and refining internal representations of expectations, then activating the other regions of the brain later. Positive expectations concerning analgesia would stimulate the dorsolateral PFC, which would then simultaneously activate the medial PFC, the orbito-frontal PFC and the opioid system of the brain (periaqueductal grey; PAG) (Fricchione et al., 2005). ACC has been postulated to attenuate pain by employing cognitive control mechanisms to modulate pain through activation of the descending opioid system via the PAG (Figure 3.10).

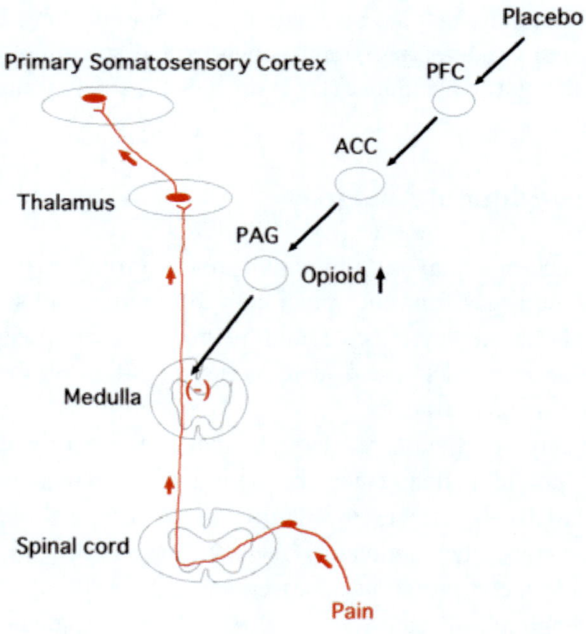

Figure 3.10. A positive expectation (placebo effects) activates endogenous opioids at the PAG through the PFC and ACC. The pain-modulating brain networks decrease the transmission along the pain pathways (red lines).

In another study of an experimental model of heat-induced pain, the neurophysiological effects of the opioid and placebo analgesics were analyzed in healthy volunteers by PET, comparing the activated areas of the brain

(Petrovic et al., 2002). Both placebo and the opioid agonist activated specific areas of the brain (medial PFC, orbito-frontal PFC and PAG) (Petrovic et al., 2002). This suggests a direct relationship between the placebo-induced analgesia and the opioid-induced analgesia.

In fMRI study, Wager et al. (2004) observed a decrease in pain with the application of a placebo cream on the arms of patients subjected to electric shocks, coinciding with an increase in brain activity in the orbito-frontal PFC, dorsolateral-medial PFC, and PAG, and decrease of brain activity in the thalamus, anterior insular cortex and ACC (Wager et al., 2004).

Similarly, spoken suggestion-induced placebo analgesia showed the decrease of neural activity in the thalamus, and ACC with a simultaneous increase in the lateral amygdale and PAG in patients with irritable bowel syndrome (IBS) (Price et al., 2007).

It has been proposed that a conviction in a positive expectation can induce a change in the activity of the PFC, whose feedback stimulates the flow of dopamine from the medial fasciculus to the ventral tegument. Receptors in the dorsal striatum (caudate nuclei and putamen), in the ventral striatum (basal nuclei) and in the prefrontal medial, orbito-frontal and dorsolateral cortices would register this tonic change in the dopamine. At the same time, activation of the PFC by positive expectation may also stimulate the opioid system of the PAG (Fricchione et al., 2005). Thus, it is highly likely that positive expectation activates endogenous opioids and pain-modulating brain networks, decreasing the transmission along the pain pathways (Figure 3.10).

4.2. Placebo Effects in IBS

A meta-analysis reviewing the placebo effect of several clinical trials for IBS in adults has found an average placebo response of 40% with a range of 16 to 71% (Patel et al., 2005). Studies on the placebo effect in adult patients with IBS showed that desires and expectations influenced placebo effects (Vase et al., 2005). Children with IBS, functional abdominal pain or FD were randomized to 4 weeks of placebo or amitriptyline (tricyclic antidepressant). The study showed that there was no significant difference in the effectiveness of amitriptyline (63%) and placebo (58%) in the treatment of these pediatric patients (Saps et al., 2009). They assumed that the high placebo effect was the result of a high level of expectancy of the subjects and the parents. In addition, a strong family-doctor relationship was observed by a frequent contact between physician and subjects throughout the study (Saps et al., 2009).

Kaptchuk et al. (2008) also demonstrated in IBS patients that the patient–practitioner relationship is probably the most robust factor contributing to the placebo effect (Kaptchuk et al., 2008). In acupuncture treatment in IBS patients, patient–practitioner relationship produced clinically significant outcomes (global improvement, adequate relief of symptoms, symptom severity score and quality of life) compared with a waiting list (neither placebo treatment nor interaction with a health care professional list) and limited interaction with a practitioner (sham acupuncture) (Kaptchuk et al., 2008).

4.3. Placebo Effects in Depression

In depression, there are clinical evidences that different regions of the brain linked to serotonin (5-HT) are involved in the placebo response for depression. The magnitude of the placebo response in the treatment of major depression was evaluated in a systematic review of 75 placebo-controlled studies. Walsh et al. (2002) demonstrated that the placebo group manifests a mean therapeutic effect of 30%, while the active group manifested 50% (Walsh et al., 2002). Similarly, the placebo effect showed a mean therapeutic response of 31 % in the placebo group, compared to 56% in the active group (Sysko et al., 2007).

Recent meta-analyses evaluation of the clinical efficacy of antidepressant medications in the treatment of major depressive disorders concluded that there was no significant difference in comparison to placebo in the patients with moderate depression, and only 'a relatively small difference for patients with very severe depression (Kirsch et al., 2008; Fournier et al., 2010).

With the objective of distinguishing the changes in brain activity caused by placebo treatment in depressive patients, Leuchter et al. (2002) conducted a clinical trial with patients suffering from major depression, who were given antidepressants or placebo for 9 weeks, then classed as 'antidepressant responsive', 'placebo-responsive', 'antidepressant non-responsive' and 'placebo non-responsive'. The correlation between the cerebral perfusion (quantified by PET) and brain activity (quantified by EEG) was also evaluated. While the pre-treatment group presented no EEG difference, the 'placebo-responsive' group manifested a significant increase of a strong correlation with the brain activity and cerebral perfusion at the PFC. This alteration was observed early in the treatment and not seen in either the 'non-responsive' group or the 'antidepressant responsive' group (Leuchter et al., 2002).

Using PET, Mayberg et al. (2002) conducted a double blind clinical trial to study the effects of anti-depressant (fluoxetine) and placebo. Remission of symptoms was observed in approximately half of each group. The placebo response was associated with an increased glucose metabolism in the PFC, parietal cortex, ACC, and PCC and decreased metabolism in the subgenual cingulate, and thalamus. Subjects who responded to fluoxetine showed a similar metabolic pattern, suggesting a possible involvement of serotonin (5-HT) in the antidepressant effects of placebo induction (Mayberg et al., 2002).

When any placebo intervention creates a positive expectation of reward, neurons of the PFC are activated by the probability of its occurrence; these cells send excitatory glutamatergic direct impulses and inhibitory GABAergic indirect impulses to the dopaminergic neurons throughout the body, with the combination of these signals being the determinant for their tonic activation. Neurons from the PFC, dorsal striatum and ventral striatum may also show tonic activation during the expectation of reward (de la Fuente-Fernandez et al., 2004).

4.4. Possible Mechanism of Placebo Effects

Central OXT seems to be involved in mediating placebo effects. As mentioned in Chapter VI, social interaction stimulates OXT release and that OXT mediates trust, analgesic and anti-depressive effects. It is conceivable that a reliable patient-doctor relationship increases OXT expression in the patients' brain, resulting in analgesic and anti-depressive effects. It remains unknown, however, whether the hypothalamic OXT stimulation is initiated via the activation of the PFC in response to a reliable patient-doctor relationship.

Enck et al. suggested that OXT is the central mediator of the placebo response and they proposed the possibility that the placebo response in trials may be predicted by circulating plasma OXT levels and/or OXT receptor density in the brain (Enck et al., 2009).

It is generally thought that placebo effects involve non-specific and/or psychological factors. However, it should be emphasized that such emotional impact (whether non-specific or psychological) can lead to beneficial effects by modulating brain activity and networking, resulting in the stimulation of various neurotransmitters and neuropeptides (opioid, OXT, 5-HT, dopamine, GABA, glutamate, etc.).

CWM has developed different kinds of agonists, such as opioid, OXT, 5-HT, dopamine, GABA, and glutamate, etc.-These drugs have been widely used to treat various diseases and symptoms. However, CWM should focus more on how to activate/upregulate the endogenous substances, rather than the exogenous administration of drugs. The development of the procedure that activates endogenous substances, which may promote the process of self-healing, is one of the most important developments for the future of medicine.

5. Autogenic Training (Auto-Suggestion)

Autogenic training is an auto-hypnotic and auto-suggestion technique. Autogenic training consists of following 6 mental exercises aimed at relieving anger, tension, and stress (Mommaerts et al., 2012).

1) Tranquility exercise to create a state of silence and concentration. Typical imagination: "I am calm. Nothing can disturb me."
2) Heaviness exercise to create a sense of heaviness in the limbs. Typical imagination: "My arms and legs are heavy."
3) Warmth exercise: to create a sense of heat in the limbs. Typical imagination: "My arms and legs are warm."
4) Breath exercise to concentrate on breathing. Typical imagination: "My breath is calm and regular."
5) Heart exercise to cause further sedation. Typical imagination: "My heart beats calmly and regularly."
6) Solar plexus exercise to deepen the relaxation. Typical imagination: "The center is warm."

Autogenic training is a psycho-physiological form of psychotherapy, which can be performed by an individual through passive concentration. Autogenic training is a therapy that is specifically aimed at stress prevention/reduction and has the advantage that once learned an individual can use it without further intervention from a therapist.

The exercises are initially taught in small groups in which patients control the feelings of warmth and heaviness, eventually gaining more and more control over autonomic functions. Autogenic training has been shown to restore the balance between activity of the sympathetic and parasympathetic branches of the autonomic nervous system with important health benefits. Patients are encouraged to perform these exercises at home on a regular basis. Autogenic training is now a popular method, advocated for controlling stress, anxiety, phobias, depression, sleep disorders, headache, pain, asthma, hypertension, etc. (Ernst et al., 2000; Kanji et al., 2006).

Motion sickness symptoms are commonly treated with intramuscular injections of promethazine. However, once healthy men received autogenic training exercise before the motion sickness tests, the motion sickness tolerance was significantly increased compared to promethazine (25 mg or 50 mg). The subjects received autogenic training exercise reported fewer or no symptoms at higher rotational velocities than subjects promethazine groups (Cowings et al., 2000).

MRI study showed that pre- and post-central cortex were significantly activated during autogenic training, compared to resting state in healthy subjects (Schlamann et al., 2010).

Mommaerts et al. (2012) proposed that the placebo effect is just one example of auto-suggestion (communication to the subconscious) and that we have to rethink much of modern regular medicine. Auto-suggestion as overt communication to the subconscious should probably be widely accepted in CWM. If this is the case, we can develop a system of auto-suggestion without the need of a placebo. There is no need for deception (Mommaerts et al., 2012).

6. Hypnosis

Hypnosis was popularly recognized in the 19th century and considered a purely psychotherapeutic intervention. Hypnotherapy has been demonstrated to have the capacity to normalize visceral sensitivity and modulate motility in the gastrointestinal (GI) tract (Prior et al., 1990a; Whorwell, 1990). Whorwell et al. reported that hypnosis treatment had specific effects that substantially improved the symptoms of irritable bowel syndrome (IBS) patients. More than 50% average reduction in IBS severity, substantial reduction in anxiety and depression, improved quality of life, and good maintenance of symptom improvement were shown after the hypnosis treatment (Whorwell et al., 1984). They also demonstrated that hypnosis is effective in the long-term management of functional dyspepsia (FD) (Calvert et al., 2002). Thus, the skills of the hypnotherapist should be made routinely available to patients with functional GI disorders.

However, the mechanism of the impact of hypnosis on functional GI disorders remains obscure. Unlike pharmaceutical agents for IBS and FD, which have a clearly delineated mechanism of action, it is largely unknown how hypnotherapy produces its effects on GI symptoms.

The capacity to increase hypnotizability (one's capacity to respond to hypnotic suggestion) has important implications. It may increase the number of people who can benefit from hypnotic interventions for psychological and medical conditions. It has been emphasized that the rapport between hypnotist and subject is pivotal to motivate the respondent to engage in strategies that allows them to suspend reality and respond to suggestions (Bryant et al., 2012).

Hypnotizability is normally distributed in the population, with approximately 15% being low hypnotizable, 70% being medium hypnotizable, and 15% being high hypnotizable (Woody et al., 2005). Increasing motivation to respond and altering the respondent's expectations modulate hypnotic responding. Hypnotic responding is enhanced by facilitating rapport by altering the hypnotherapist's behavior (Sheehan, 1980).

6.1. Possible Mechanism of Hypnosis

OXT released in response to social stimuli may be part of a neuroendocrine substrate, which underlies the benefits of positive social experiences. Such processes may explain the health-promoting effects of certain alternative therapies. Because of the special properties of OXT, including the fact that it can become conditioned to psychological state or imagery, OXT may mediate the benefits attributed to hypnosis therapy (Uvnas-Moberg et al., 2005). OXT administration, which enhances social bonding in humans, may enhance hypnotic responding. When low hypnotizable individuals were administered OXT via nasal spray, their level of hypnotic responding increased significantly (Bryant et al., 2012).

7. Homeopathy

Homeopathy was developed more than 200 years ago by Samuel Hahnemann. It is based on the principles that a disease can be cured by a substance that produces similar symptoms in healthy people. In order to minimize the possible aggravations of original treatment, homeopathy is believed to reduce the primary effects of medication and develop its 'latent dynamic' power, by the serial dilution with succession (Jong et al., 2012).

To increase the probability of success in the choice of individualized medicine, the homeopathic physician takes an individualizing history by asking the patient to describe various classes of symptomatic manifestations. This process of individualization is a gradual one and may require a prolonged observation period, with follow-up and different prescriptions, until the ideal medication is achieved.

The effects of medical treatment can be divided into specific and non-specific. The specific effects are the direct physiological or pharmacological effects and non-specific effects are all other components of the treatment process. It has been argued that, whatever the specific effects of homeopathic medicines, the homeopathic intervention as a whole is of benefit, due to factors including the in-depth consultation and careful attention to the individual case (Weatherley-Jones et al., 2004). It is widely assumed that the homeopathic consultation is itself of benefit. However, the relative contribution of specific and non-specific factors in homeopathic treatment is unknown. A definitive trial of the design is unlikely to discriminate the relative contributions of the non-specific and specific effects to the outcome of homeopathic treatment of dermatitis, because of patient preference issues (Fisher et al., 2006)

The non-specific therapeutic effects of the doctor–patient relationship are likely to be increased by the patient's expectations of the homeopathic method which meshes with the specific therapeutic effects of the medicines (Teixeira et al., 2010). It remains to be investigated whether homeopathic treatment may utilize brain activation and networks in the same way as placebo.

SUMMARY

Various types of meditation techniques, including Yoga, Tai-chi, Qi-gong, Zen and LKM, improve psychological disorders (anxiety and depression), pain syndromes, and cardiovascular symptoms. It is conceivable that the beneficial effects of these procedures on pain reduction are mediated via the activation of PFC/ACC and stimulation of opioid release from the PAG (Figure 3.11).

Prolonged stress exposure causes malfunctioning of the PFC. Anti-stress effect is mediated via the activation of PFC/ACC and stimulation of OXT release from the PVN. It is likely that placebo, hypnosis and auto-suggestion also utilize the similar pathways with the meditation. In addition, these mind-body therapies may adjust the imbalance of autonomic nerves function associated with stress (Figure 3.12).

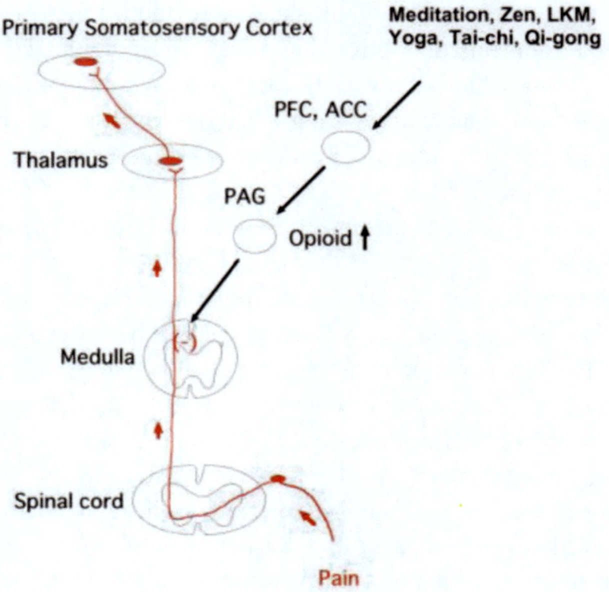

Figure 3.11. PFC and ACC are activated by meditation, Zen, LKM, Yoga, Tai-chi, and Qi-gong, which can stimulate opioid release from the PAG, resulting in pain reduction.

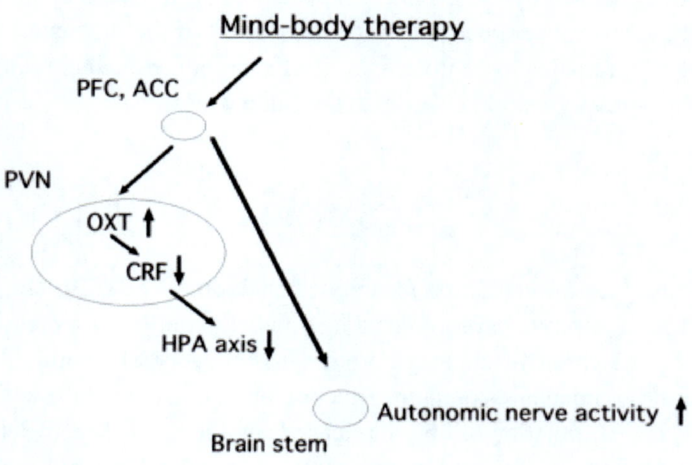

Figure 3.12. Mind-body therapies including meditation, placebo, hypnosis, and auto-suggestion activate PFC and ACC, which can stimulate OXT release form the PVN. Activated PFC and ACC may also regulate autonomic nerve function.

Chapter 4

MANUAL THERAPIES

Complementary and alternative medicine (CAM) therapies include acupuncture, massage, chiropractic, aromatherapy, music therapy, etc. The beneficial effects of these therapies are, at least in part, due to stimulation of sensory neurons in our body. It has been demonstrated that somatic afferents from the skin and muscle are involved in the control of autonomic functions in animals (Sato et al., 1975; Kametani et al., 1979; Koizumi et al., 1980) and humans (Camilleri et al., 1984).

Electrical stimulation of the sciatic nerve inhibited intestinal motility via the activation of splanchnic nerves in dogs (Lehman, 1913). Sensory stimulation of the abdominal skin inhibited gastric motility via increasing gastric sympathetic nerve activity in rats (Sato et al., 1975; Koizumi et al., 1980). In contrast, pinching the hind paw enhanced gastric motility by exciting gastric vagal nerve activity (Kametani et al., 1979). In healthy humans, transcutaneous electrical nerve stimulation (TENS) applied to the hand and abdomen reduced antral motility (Camilleri et al., 1984). These studies provide good evidence indicating the importance of cutaneous input in autonomic control of gastrointestinal (GI) functions.

1. SOMATOSENSORY PATHWAY

Somatic sensation comprises of four main modalities, each relaying tactile, thermal, painful, or pruritic (itch) information to the central nervous system (CNS). These input channels can be further classified as subserving a sensory function of spatial and temporal localization, discrimination, and provision of essential information for controlling and guiding exploratory tactile behaviors.

Sensory axons are classified according to their degree of myelination, the fatty sheath that surrounds the nerve fiber. The degree of myelination determines the speed with which the axon can conduct nerve impulses and hence the nerves' conduction velocity. Human discriminative tactile sensibility is solely mediated by large myelinated afferents. However, a further subtype of afferent slowly conducting unmyelinated C-fibers exists in human hairy skin that are neither nociceptive nor pruritic, but that respond preferentially to low force, slowly moving mechanical stimuli traversing their receptive fields.

The largest and fastest axons are called A-alpha and include some of the proprioceptive neurons, such as the muscle stretch receptors. The second largest group, called A-beta, includes all of the discriminative touch receptors. Pain, itch, and temperature include the third and fourth groups, A-delta and C-fibers (Wilson et al., 2009).

The spinal–supraspinal pathways responsible for somatosensory stimulation mainly comprise the posterior spinal cord column pathway and the spinothalamic pathway. Most peripheral thick myelinated afferent fibers (A-alpha and A-beta fibers) activated by the discriminative touch and sense of vibration enter the ipsilateral dorsal column-medial lemniscus tract (posterior column pathway) and emerge into the contalateral spinothalamic pathway. In contrast, the thinly myelinated or unmyelinated afferent fibers (A-delta and C-fibers) activated by pain and temperature are carried up by the contalateral spinothalamic tract to supraspinal levels (spinothalamic pathway). These impulses are further relayed to the thalamus, and ultimately sent to the primary somatosensory cortex (Hendelman et al., 2010) (Figure 4.1).

2. Skin Contact (Touch)

Tactile C-afferents have a unique and different primary function compared with the myelinated afferents. An essential role of the tactile C-afferents is to convey information to limbic structures of light skin deformation, which may promote a pleasant feeling of touch as a counterpart to the unpleasant feelings associated with painful stimuli (Wessberg et al., 2003).

The soft touches that arise from the gentler sweeping movements common during grooming may activate a class of unmyelinated afferent fibers (C-fibers) that project to both the limbic system and the orbito-frontal cortex (Francis et al., 1999; Olausson et al., 2002). This route is quite distinct from the more conventional somatosensory routes (touch, pain, heat and itch) that underpin discriminative touch sensation involve low threshold mechanoreceptors in the skin and large diameter A-beta fibers projecting to the sensory cortex. In contrast, the unmyelinated c-fibers appear to give rise to a pleasant sensation of light touch when skin is stroked lightly (McGlone et al., 2007; Dunbar, 2010).

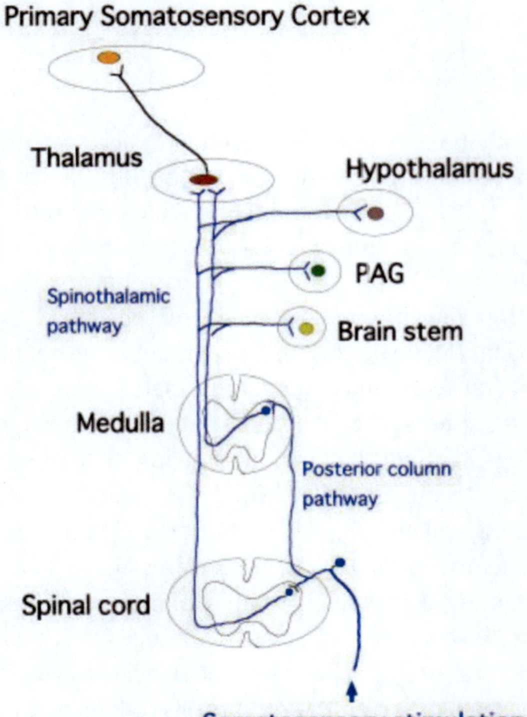

Figure 4.1. The spinal–supraspinal pathways responsible for somatosensory stimulation comprise the posterior spinal cord column pathway and the spinothalamic pathway. These impulses are further relayed to the thalamus (blue lines), and ultimately sent to the primary somatosensory cortex (a black line). In addition, somatosensory impulses are relayed to other brain areas, including the brain stem, PAG, and hypothalamus via collateral connections (blue lines).

It has been demonstrated that pleasant touch gives rise to a different activation pattern in the human brain than neutral touch, notably activation of an area in the orbito-frontal cortex close to areas responding to pleasant taste and smell (Francis et al., 1999). In functional magnetic resonance imaging (fMRI) study, pleasant touch to the hand with velvet produced stronger activation of the orbito-frontal cortex than affectively neutral touch of the hand with wood. In contrast, the affectively neutral but more intense touch produced more activation of the primary somatosensory cortex than the pleasant stimulus. This indicates that part of the orbito-frontal cortex is concerned with representing the positively affective aspects of somatosensory stimuli (Francis et al., 1999).

2.1. Touch and Social Life

A light touch stimulus, which was slowly moving over the hairy skin of the forearm, produced a strong activation of the insular cortex. Thus, the essential role of the C-afferents system is to provide emotional and behavioral responses to affiliative or friendly skin-to-skin contact (Olausson et al., 2002; Wessberg et al., 2003).

In primates, grooming is a major feature of social life. Grooming is all about physical touch (Dunbar, 2010). For primates, grooming is a social activity whose function seems to be mainly associated with social bonding. An animal that is being groomed can become relaxed. Social grooming has a number of physiological effects that include slowing of heart rate and lowering behavioral indices of stress (Dunbar, 2010).

Having grooming relationships can buffer a female against stressful challenges. In baboons, during a socially stressful event, females who responded by contacting their social network exhibited a significantly faster reduction in cortisol levels than females who did not focus their grooming on core partners. Thus, it seems that female baboons can enhance their sense of security, with consequent amelioration of physiological stress levels by grooming (Wittig et al., 2008). Keverne et al. (1989) have shown that grooming increases the production of endorphin in the groomee, suggesting that brain opioids may play an important role in mediating social attachment. An essential role of grooming is to promote affectionate attachment between individuals, and to keep the group together (Keverne et al., 1989).

In humans, blood pressure is sensitive to supportive and non-supportive interactions between partners (Broadwell et al., 1999; Grewen et al., 2003). Emotional support and affection in couples is expressed through physical touch, such as hand-holding, hugs, and sitting- or lying- cuddled up (Grewen et al., 2003).

In women, the frequency of physical contact (hugs) with partners was correlated with lower blood pressure (Light et al., 2005). It has been shown that enhanced oxytocin (OXT) activity is one of the primary physiological mediators of the health benefits of emotional support, particularly those linked to warm touch (Carter, 1998; Uvnas-Moberg, 1998b) (See Chapter VII). The frequent hugs between spouses/partners were associated with lower blood pressure and higher plasma OXT levels (Light et al., 2005).

3. Acupuncture

Acupuncture has been in practice in China for over 3,000 years and used for treating various GI diseases, including gastroparesis, functional dyspepsia (FD), irritable bowel syndrome (IBS), constipation and diarrhea (Chang et al., 2001; Wang, 2004; Takahashi, 2006; Tillisch, 2006). Acupuncture has also been used for the treatment of cardiovascular diseases, metabolic diseases, chronic pain, mood disorders, etc.

According to traditional Chinese medicine concepts, the energy force, known as *Qi*, runs through the body. *Qi* energy enters the body through specific acupuncture points and flows to deeper organ structures, bringing life-giving nourishment of a subtle energetic nature. Meridians are classified on the basis of the direction in which *Qi* flows on the surface of the body. If the flow of *Qi* is insufficient, or interrupted, *Yin* and *Yang* become unbalanced and illness may occur (Helms, 1998). However, the ancient concept of *Qi* and meridians has no counterpart in modern studies of chemistry, biology, and physics.

Acupuncture is believed to restore the balance of *Yin* and *Yang*. Acupuncture loci, also known as acupoints, are the skin needling points used for acupuncture treatment. In humans, more than 300 acupoints are located along the meridians. Acupoints are thought to be specific points reflecting visceral conditions and organs (Melzack et al., 1977) (Figure 4.2). Despite the fact that specific acupoints are used for treating specific symptoms and/or diseases, it is not fully understood how their specificity is determined and how the needling at acupoints works.

Ahn et al. (2008) conducted a systematic review of studies directly evaluating the electrical characteristics of acupuncture structures and appropriate controls. There was no clear evidence to demonstrate the existence of acupuncture points or meridians (Ahn et al., 2008).

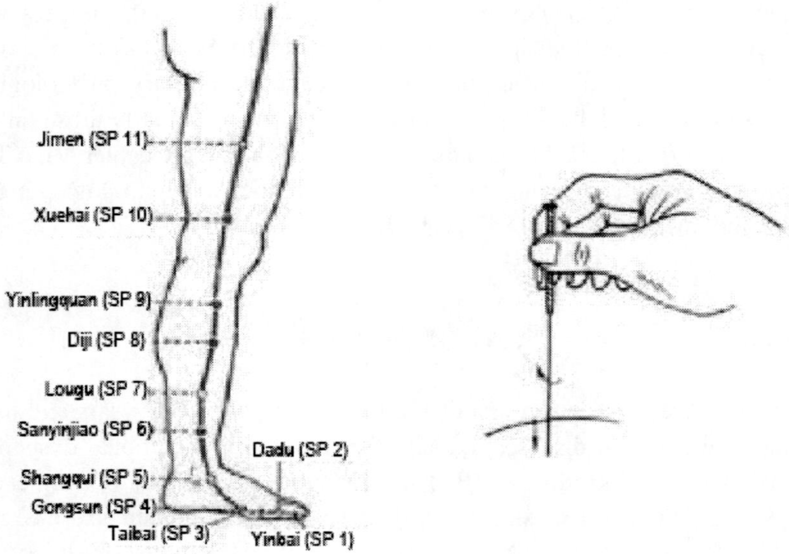

Figure 4.2. Acupuncture points (left) and manual stimulation technique (right).

3.1. Possible Mechanisms of Acupuncture

In order to be widely accepted by both patients and physicians, the beneficial effects of acupuncture should be proven by our Western medicine terminology and methodologies. Acupuncture treatment involves the insertion of thin needles into the skin and underlying muscle layer. In a traditional acupuncture procedure, the inserted needles are twisted right and left at 0.5-1 second intervals. Recently, acupuncture needles are stimulated by electricity under various frequencies of 1-100 Hz (electro-acupuncture; EA). Thus, the procedure may stimulate the somatic afferent nerves of the skin and muscles.

As described above, the spinal–supraspinal pathways responsible for somatosensory stimulation mainly comprise the posterior spinal cord column pathway and the spinothalamic pathway. These impulses are further relayed to the thalamus, and ultimately sent to the primary somatosensory cortex. In addition, somatosensory impulses are relayed to other brain areas, including the brain stem, periaqueductal gray (PAG), and hypothalamus, via collateral connections (Hendelman et al., 2010) (Figure 4.1).

The nucleus tractus solitarius (NTS) is the primary brain stem relay for visceral information from cardiovascular, respiratory and GI systems. In addition, recent studies indicate that the NTS also receives somatic afferent inputs (Menetrey et al., 1987; Gamboa-Esteves et al., 2001). Electrophysiological study demonstrated that the NTS receives input from low- and high-threshold cutaneous mechanoreceptors. NTS neurons are activated by the rhythmic and sustained muscle stretch of the hind limb (Toney et al., 2000). Neurons of the NTS and the spinal cord were labeled by injection of neuroanatomical tracers to the acupoints of hind limb (Stomach-36; ST-36) in rats (Lee et al., 2001a).

C-Fos is a cellular proto-oncogene belonging to the immediate early gene family of transcription factors. Once neurons are activated, c-fos expression is upregulated. By immunohistochemistry of c-Fos, the location of activated neurons can easily be detected. Acupuncture at the facial acupoints increases the number of c-Fos immunopositive cells in the NTS in rats (Liu et al., 2004a). Therefore, it is highly likely that somatic stimulation induced by acupuncture is conveyed to the NTS.

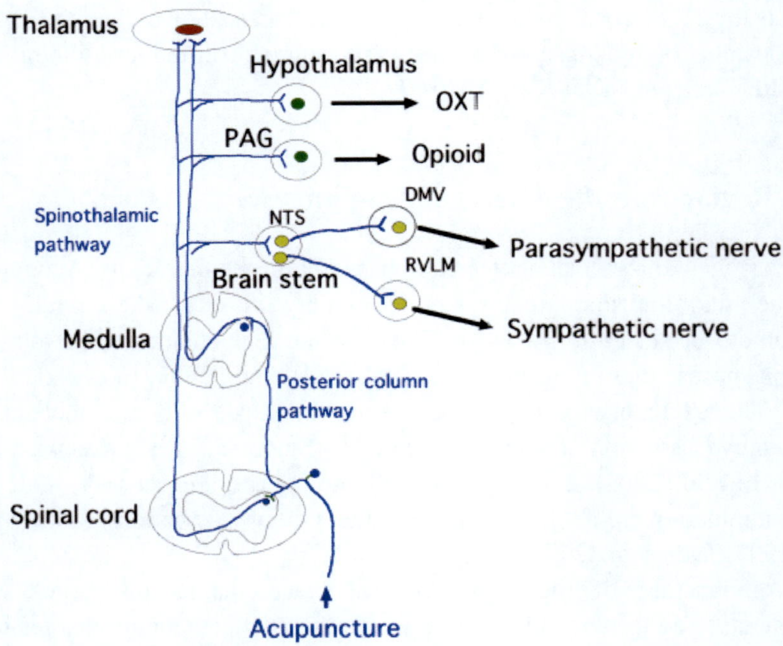

Figure 4.3. NTS neurons at the brain stem are stimulated by acupuncture. Then, autonomic nerve function is altered via the activation of the DMV and RVLM. Acupuncture also activates the PAG and hypothalamus, resulting in the release of opioid and OXT, respectively.

The NTS is adjacent to the dorsal motor nucleus of vagi (DMV) and both compose the dorsal vagal complex (DVC). The DVC integrates vago-vagal reflex, which plays a major role in regulation of GI motor function (Travagli et al., 1992; Washabau et al., 1995). The NTS neurons also project to the rostral ventrolateral medulla (RVLM) of the brain stem (Agarwal et al., 1991; Suzuki et al., 1997; Kantzides et al., 2005). The RVLM neurons provide drive to the sympathetic preganglionic neurons in the intermediolateral nucleus of the spinal cord (Laskey et al., 1988). When NTS neurons are stimulated by acupuncture, autonomic nerve function is altered via the activation of the DMV and/or RVLM (Figure 4.3).

In addition to the NTS, DMV and RVLM, acupuncture may activate some other nuclei in the brain. EA at pericardium-6 (PC-6; hand) activates neurons in the arcuate nucleus (ARC) and PAG and inhibits the activity of RVLM, suggesting the existence of ARC-PAG-RVLM neuronal pathway. This pathway may mediate EA inhibition on visceral excitatory cardiovascular reflexes (Li et al., 2009). Similar mechanisms might be utilized to produce the effects of EA on GI motor function. It has been shown that the PAG is responsible for mu receptor agonist- and neurotensin-induced inhibition of intestinal transit (Tache et al., 1990).

3.2. Region-Specific Effects of Acupuncture

It is well known that acupuncture has region specific effects. Acupuncture of the hind limbs stimulates gastric motility in rats (Sato et al., 1993; Fukumoto et al., 2003; Li et al., 2007), while acupuncture of the abdomen inhibits gastric motility (Sato et al., 1993; Tada et al., 2003; Li et al., 2007) in rats. The excitatory gastric responses to the hind limb are abolished by vagotomy (dissection of vagus nerve) in rats (Sato et al., 1993; Tatewaki et al., 2003; Li et al., 2007). In contrast, the inhibitory gastric responses to abdominal skin stimulation are abolished by sympathetic nerve dissection in rats (Sato et al., 1993; Tada et al., 2003).

Acupuncture of the hind limbs increases vagus discharges, while acupuncture on the abdominal surface increases sympathetic discharges in rats (Sato et al., 1993; Li et al., 2007).

Sympathetic and parasympathetic activity can be evaluated by heart rate variability (HRV) analysis in conscious animals non-invasively. The power in the high frequency (HF) band of HRV represents parasympathetic activities in rats (Kuwahara et al., 1994; Imai et al., 2009) and humans (Pomeranz et al.,

1985). In contrast, the power in the low frequency (LF) band of HRV represents sympathetic activities in rats (Kuwahara et al., 1994; Imai et al., 2009) and a combination of sympathetic and parasympathetic activities in humans (Pomeranz et al., 1985), respectively. EA at ST-36 decreases, while EA at stomach-25 (ST-25; abdomen) increases the ratio of LF/HF in normal rats (Imai et al., 2008), suggesting that inhibitory gastric responses to the abdomen are mediated via sympathetic nerves. In contrast, the excitatory gastric responses to the hind limb are mediated via the vagus nerves.

EA at ST-36 increases the number of c-Fos immunopositive cells at the DMV and the caudal part of the NTS, while EA at ST-25 increases the number of c-Fos immunopositive cells at the RVLM and medio-caudal part of the NTS in rats. This suggests that somatic afferents activated by EA at ST-36 is conveyed to the caudal NTS and stimulates the DMV neurons. In contrast, somatic afferents activated by EA at ST-25 is conveyed to the medio-caudal NTS and stimulates the RVLM neurons (Iwa et al., 2007). Thus, EA at ST-25 inhibits gastric motility via the somatosensory–NTS–RVLM- sympathetic efferent pathway. In contrast, EA at ST-36 stimulates gastric motility via the somatosensory–NTS–DMV– parasympathetic efferent pathway (Figure 4.3). Thus, its neuronal pathway can explain the region-specific effects of acupuncture.

3.3. Western Medical Acupuncture

White (2009) recently proposed the modern definition of acupuncture, “Western medical acupuncture” (White, 2009). Western medical acupuncture is a therapeutic modality involving the insertion of fine needles; it is an adaptation of Chinese acupuncture using current knowledge of anatomy, physiology and pathology. The term "Western medical acupuncture" is used to distinguish it from acupuncture used as part of Chinese traditional medicine.

Western medical acupuncture regards acupuncture as part of conventional medicine rather than a complete alternative medicine. Conventional healthcare practitioners currently use western medical acupuncture, most commonly in primary care. It is mainly used to treat musculoskeletal pain, including myofascial trigger point pain. Practitioners of Western medical acupuncture tend to pay less attention than classical Chinese acupuncturists on choosing one point over another, while classical Chinese acupuncturists generally choose classical points as the best places to stimulate the nervous system (White, 2009).

3.3.1. Trigger Points vs Acupuncture Points

A myofascial trigger point is defined as a localized, hyperirritable nodule nested within a palpable taut band of skeletal muscle or fascia. Trigger point injections with local anesthetics have been performed to alleviate musculoskeletal pain since the early 1930s. No significant differences in subjective pain have been reported when comparing the effects of lidocaine injection with "dry needle stimulation" of trigger points. This suggests that the site-specific needling of the trigger point may be exclusively responsible for the observed anti-nociceptive effects (Hong, 1994; Srbely et al., 2010).

Sensitized nociceptors might be a possible cause of localized tenderness, referred pain, and local twitch response. Myofascial active trigger points are supposed to be sites where nociceptors, such as polymodaltype receptors, have been sensitized by various factors. The trigger point insertion of the needle (but not always acupuncture point insertion) affects sensitized nociceptors. Thus, dry needle stimulation of myofascial active trigger points produces greater activation of sensitized polymodaltype receptors, resulting in greater pain relief (Itoh et al., 2012). The practitioners of Western medical acupuncture use classical points (acupuncture points; acupoints) based on the assumption that they are probably optimal for sensory stimulation of the nervous system. More attention is focused on the tissue level and the type and amount of stimulation given (White, 2009).

Thus, it is conceivable to say that the effective points have been named differently; trigger points in CWM and acupoints in TCM. Trigger points associated with myofascial and visceral pains often lie within the areas of referred pain but many are located at a distance from them. When compared for spatial distribution and pain referral patterns, Melzack et al. (1977) demonstrated a remarkable 71% correlation between trigger points and acupoints (Melzack et al., 1977). Although discovered independently and labeled differently, this close correlation suggests the same underlying neural mechanisms.

3.3.2. Circulation of Qi vs Neuromodulation

Acupuncture, which has been practiced in China for over 3,000 years, involves the site-specific application of needles to specific points (acupoints) on the body to evoke a broad range of systematic therapeutic effects. Historical nomenclature describes acupoints as distinct anatomic coordinates lying along parallel longitudinal arrays of energy (*Qi*) channels (meridians) in the body. Needle stimulation of these points is believed to facilitate the flow of

Qi along these meridians; however, this concept is still under scientific observation and examination.

Western medical acupuncture no longer adheres to concepts such as *Yin/Yang* and circulation of *Qi*. Western medical acupuncture acts mainly by stimulating the nervous system, and its known modes of action include local anti-dromic axon reflexes, segmental and extra-segmental neuromodulation, and other CNS effects (White, 2009; Srbely et al., 2010). It has been shown that electrical stimulation of peripheral nerves (tibial nerve and sciatic nerve) results in an inhibition to the pain pathways at the spinal cord level in cats (Hanai, 2000). The needle insertion into trigger points, not acupuncture points, also affects sensitized nociceptors (Itoh et al., 2012).

Trigger point acupuncture provides significantly more relief on chronic low back pain and neck pain as compared with standard acupuncture (Itoh et al., 2004; Itoh et al., 2007) but not of chronic knee pain (Tough et al., 2009). These findings suggest that the myofascial pain near joints in contrast to other types of chronic pain may depend on different factors such as inflammation and joint pain. Therefore, the effects of standard acupuncture on chronic myofascial pain may be as effective as trigger point acupuncture (Itoh et al., 2012).

3.4. Analgesic (Anti-Nociceptive) Effects of Acupuncture

Opioid neurons play an important role to reduce painful sensation (analgesic effects or anti-nociceptive effects). Nociceptive messages from the spinal cord to the brain are suppressed by the descending inhibition system. Opioid neurons at the PAG play an important role of descending inhibition (Millan, 2002).

It has been well demonstrated that the analgesic effects of acupuncture are mediated by an endogenous opioid pathway (Stux et al., 1995; Diehl, 1999). The painful sensation induced by rectal distension is attenuated by EA at ST-36 in dogs. Naloxone is a non-selective antagonist of opioid receptors. The anti-nociceptive effect of EA at ST-36 is abolished by pretreatment with naloxone hydrochloride, a drug that can across the blood-brain barrier (BBB), but not naloxone methiodide, which does not cross the BBB. This suggests that EA at ST-36 reduces visceral pain via a central opioid pathway (Iwa et al., 2005).

Opioid-induced anti-nociception is mediated by the pathway from PAG to various brain nuclei. Opioids are likely to exert direct effects on PAG projection neurons through both delta- and mu-opioid receptors (Wang et al., 2002a). EA can induce the expression of opioid peptides and opioid receptors in the CNS (Gao et al., 1997; Guo et al., 1997). EA attenuates visceral hypersensitivity in rat IBS model (Wu et al., 2008). Using a double immunohistochemistry of c-Fos and enkephalin, Dr. Longhurst's group showed that EA activated opioid neurons at the PAG in cats (Guo et al., 2004; Guo et al., 2007) (Figure 4.3).

Using fMRI, acupuncture-induced modulation of CNS activity can be studied non-invasively in humans, allowing for comparison to animal studies. The PAG and cortical areas responds to manual acupuncture at Large Intestine-4 (LI-4; hand), while sham-acupuncture results in reduced levels of the PAG and cortical activity (Liu et al., 2004b). Activation in the ventrolateral PAG is greater for EA at ST-36, compared to sham EA (Napadow et al., 2009). The PAG and cortical areas respond to manual acupuncture of the hand (Liu et al., 2004b).

As mentioned above, EA has an anti-nociceptive effect via central opioid release. Viscero-motor response (VMR) to colorectal distension was attenuated by EA in rats (Gao et al., 1997; Guo et al., 1997; Wu et al., 2008). As EA activate PAG neurons (Guo et al., 2004; Guo et al., 2007), it is conceivable that EA impulses are relayed via collateral connections to the PAG, which contains the endogenous opioids. PAG sends inhibitory information to the spinal dorsal horn and blocks noxious signal inputs from the periphery (descending inhibition) (Figure 4.4, #1). Hanai (2000) showed that electrical stimulation of peripheral nerves results in an inhibition to the pain pathways at the spinal cord level in cats (Hanai, 2000). This suggests another possibility that acupuncture may inhibit the pain pathway at the spinal cord levels (Figure 4.4, #2).

In addition to opioids, it has been shown that hypothalamic OXT has anti-nociceptive effects (Stock et al., 1988; Uvnas-Moberg et al., 1993; Agren et al., 1995; Yang et al., 2007) (See Chapter VII). As mentioned earlier, somatosensory simulation is carried to the hypothalamus as well (Figure 4.1). A recent study showed that EA can stimulate OXT expression at the PVN (Yoshimoto et al., 2012a) (Figure 4.3), indicating that anti-nociceptive effect of acupuncture is mediated by the combined actions of opioid and OXT.

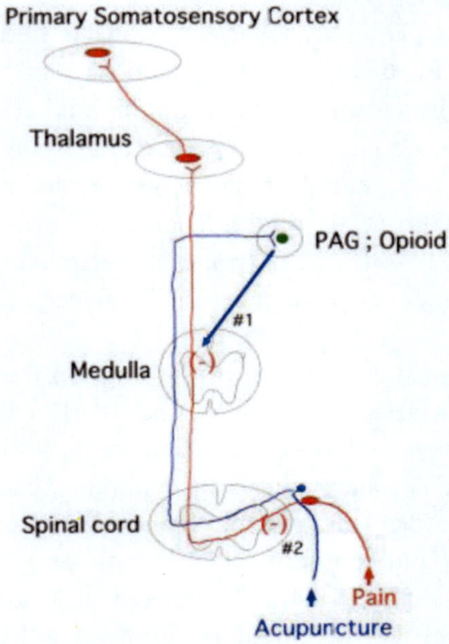

Figure 4.4. Acupuncture stimulate opioid release from the PAG (blue lines). Released opioid blocks noxious signal inputs from the periphery at the spinal dorsal horn **(#1)**. Acupuncture also inhibits the pain pathway (red lines) at the spinal cord levels **(#2)**.

3.5. Anti-Emetic Effects of Acupuncture

Acupoint of PC-6 (hand) has been used for nausea and vomiting. PC-6 is located in the groove caudal to the flexor carpi radialis and cranial to the superficial digital flexor muscles. In 1987, Dundee et al. reported that acupuncture at PC-6 decreases cisplatin-associated nausea and vomiting (Dundee et al., 1987). A clinical study also demonstrated that EA at PC-6 significantly inhibits the postoperative nausea and vomiting after the surgery (Dundee et al., 1989; Gan et al., 2004). EA at PC-6 reduces motion sickness in healthy volunteers (Hu et al., 1992; Lin et al., 1997).

Level of plasma vasopressin is rapidly elevated in response to diverse emetic stimuli such as motion stimuli (Kim et al., 1997) and anti-cancer drugs (Edwards et al., 1989; Cubeddu et al., 1990). Intravenous injection of vasopressin results in vomiting and retching in humans (Rowe et al., 1979; Kim et al., 1997) and dogs (Carpenter et al., 1984; Chen et al., 2003). Acupuncture at ST-36 and PC-6 attenuates symptom scores of emesis induced by vasopressin infusion in dogs (Chen et al., 2003). Retrograde propulsive movement of GI tract is highly associated with the frequency of retching and vomiting. EA at PC-6 reduces the frequency of retrograde propulsive movement induced by vasopressin in dogs (Tatewaki et al., 2005).

Opioids have dual effects: an anti-emetic effect as well as an emetic effect. It has been shown that central opioid plays a major role in mediating anti-emetic effect (Costello et al., 1977). The emetic effect is mediated via the chemoreceptor trigger zone (CTZ), whereas the anti-emetic effect is mediated via the vomiting center (Costello et al., 1977; Blancquaert et al., 1986; Foss et al., 1998).

The CTZ is contained in the area postrema on the caudal margin of the forth ventricles. As area postrema has no BBB, naloxone methiodide (a peripheral opioid antagonist) can antagonize the emetic effect of opioid mediated via the CTZ. In contrast, the vomiting center is deeply located beneath the solitary tract of the caudal brain stem. Both the emetic and anti-emetic effects of opioid can be blocked by naloxone, because naloxone can cross the BBB (Foss et al., 1998). Naloxone hydrochloride, but not naloxone methiodide, abolishes the anti-emetic effect of EA at PC-6 in dogs (Tatewaki et al., 2005). This suggests that the anti-emetic effect of EA at PC-6 is mediated via the central opioid pathway.

3.6. Anti-Stress Effects of Acupuncture

Animal studies demonstrate that TENS or EA alter various stress-induced physiological responses (Han et al., 1999; Li et al., 2001; Yang et al., 2002; Manni et al., 2009). Delayed gastric emptying and accelerated colonic transit induced by acute restraint stress were restored by EA, performed on the hind limbs (ST-36) in rats (Iwa et al., 2006). The occurrence of gastric interdigestive contractions was almost completely abolished by acoustic stress in conscious dogs. EA at ST-36 significantly restored the inhibitory effects of acoustic stress on gastric interdigestive contractions (Taniguchi et al., 2012).

Heart rate and LF component were increased in response to restraint stress in rats (Imai et al., 2009) and acoustic stress in dogs (Taniguchi et al., 2012), suggesting increased activity of sympathetic tone during the stress loading. EA at ST-36 attenuated the elevated LF component and increased the HF component in response to stress in rats (Imai et al., 2009) and dogs (Taniguchi et al., 2012). These suggest that EA at ST-36 stimulates parasympathetic activity and inhibits sympathetic activity under the stressful conditions, resulting in the restoration of impaired gastric motility.

As described in Chapter VII, central OXT has anti-stress effects via inhibiting CRF expression at the PVN. The anti-stress effects of acupuncture are also mediated via the stimulation of hypothalamic OXT expression. Yoshimoto et al. (2012) recently showed EA increased the number of OXT-immunopositive cells and decreased CRF-immunopositive cells at the PVN following chronic stress (Yoshimoto et al., 2012a) (Figure 4.5). These suggest that EA may act on OXT neurons at the PVN, resulting in reduced CRF expression and HPA axis following chronic stress (Figure 4.6). Others also showed that EA reduced CRF expression at the hypothalamus in rat IBS model (Ma et al., 2009).

In humans, post-traumatic stress disorders (PTSD) are marked by deficits in anxiety, stress regulation and in social functioning. A recent clinical trial demonstrated that acupuncture is effective for treating the patients with PTSD. People diagnosed with PTSD were randomized to either an empirically developed acupuncture treatment or a group cognitive-behavioral therapy. Compared with the cognitive-behavioral therapy, acupuncture provided significant effects on PTSD. Symptom reductions observed at the time when acupuncture treatments ended, were maintained at 3-month follow-up (Hollifield et al., 2007).

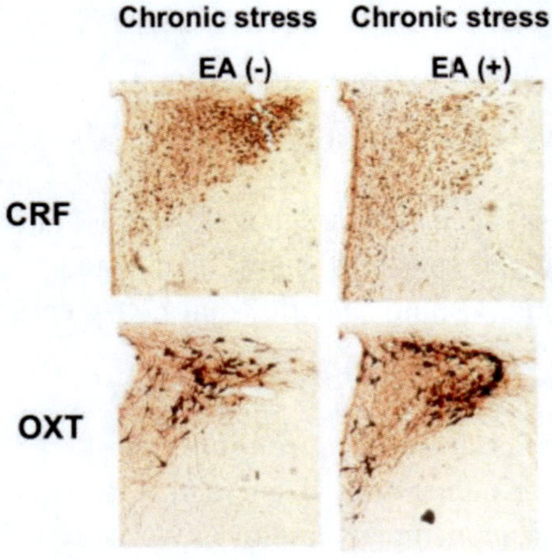

Adopted from Yoshimoto et al. (2012b).

Figure 4.5. Effects of EA on CRF and OXT expression at the PVN following chronic stress in rats.

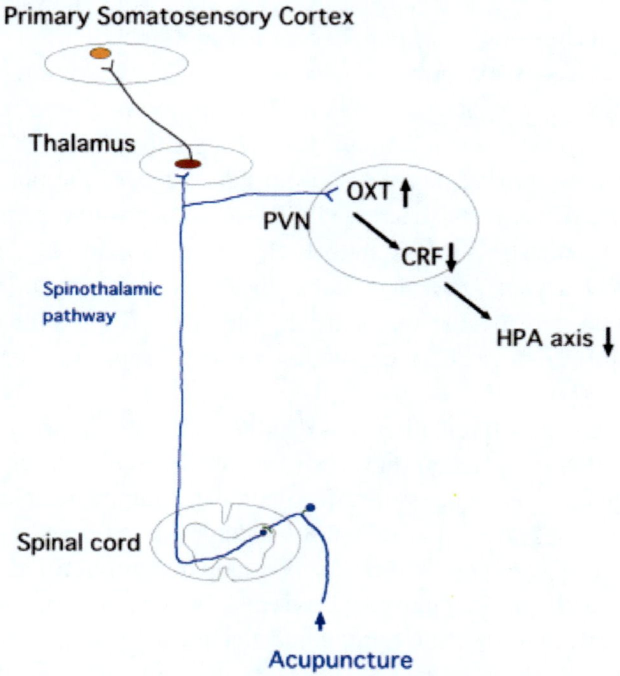

Figure 4.6. Acupuncture acts on OXT neurons at the PVN (blue lines), resulting in reduced CRF expression and HPA axis following chronic stress.

3.7. Placebo Effects of Acupuncture

Clinical studies suggested that both specific and non-specific factors might play a role in acupuncture therapy. Some studies of acupuncture, with the objective of distinguishing specific from non-specific therapeutic effects, have been reported.

3.7.1. Sham Acupuncture vs Real Acupuncture

There have been numerous evidences that real (active) acupuncture is superior than sham acupuncture in cardiovascular function (Flachskampf et al., 2007; McFadden et al., 2010), postoperative pain (Sun et al., 2008b), headache (Sun et al., 2008a), neck and low back pain (Furlan et al.). These studies suggest that the placebo effects (non-specific effects) are minor for acupuncture treatment.

Ezzo et al. (2000) searched and reviewed the effectiveness of acupuncture for chronic pain. Trials were included if they were randomized, had populations with pain longer than 3 months. Results were positive in 21 studies, negative in 3 and neutral in 27. High-quality studies clustered in designs using sham acupuncture as the control group. Six or more acupuncture treatments were significantly associated with positive outcomes. They concluded there is limited evidence that acupuncture is more effective than no treatment for chronic pain; and inconclusive evidence that acupuncture is more effective than placebo, sham acupuncture or standard care (Ezzo et al., 2000).

Others reviewed the randomized trials longer than 6 weeks in duration that compared needle acupuncture with a sham, usual care, or waiting list control group for patients with knee osteoarthritis. Sham-controlled trials show clinically irrelevant short-term benefits of acupuncture for treating knee osteoarthritis. Waiting list-controlled trials suggest clinically relevant benefits, some of which may be due to placebo or expectation effects (Manheimer et al., 2007). Similarly, no statistically significant differences were observed between acupuncture and sham acupuncture, but both groups had significant reductions in pain compared with the waiting group (Suarez-Almazor et al., 2010).

In sham acupuncture procedure, needles are generally inserted into the non-meridian points, while needles are inserted into the meridian points in real acupuncture based on the traditional Chinese medicine. As described in Chapter I, however, the meridian system has not been proved by our modern science. On the other hand, recent anatomical and physiological studies demonstrated an important role of somatosensory pathway to mediate anti-nociceptive effects and autonomic function. Therefore, it is conceivable that the somatosensory stimulation on the non-meridian points may have similar effects with the somatosensory stimulation on the meridian points. Acupuncture often shows only a small positive trend compared to sham needling, but this may be explained that these studies are simply comparing two forms of somatosensory stimulation.

3.7.2. Psychological Factors

The psychological factors (often referred to as placebo) become particularly important, because psychological factors rely on the endogenous modulation of various functions. Acupuncture is possibly a uniquely effective method in the activation of positive placebo effects.

The analgesic effects of acupuncture and placebo were compared in different painful conditions (migraine, chronic low back pain and osteoarthritis). Patients who believed they were in acupuncture group showed clinical improvements superior to those who believed they were in the placebo group (Bausell et al., 2005). Patients with high expectations about the effects of acupuncture showed more response than those who did not believe in the treatment, independently of treatment group (Linde et al., 2007).

The patients with IBS were divided into 3 groups: (1) waiting list (assessment and observation), (2) placebo acupuncture alone (limited interaction with a practitioner), and (3) placebo acupuncture with a patient–practitioner relationship (augmented by warmth, attention and confidence). The 3 groups manifested significant, progressive and similar improvements in the outcomes (Kaptchuk et al., 2008). The percentage of patients reporting adequate relief (62% and 61% at 3 and 6 weeks, respectively) is comparable with the responder rate in clinical trials of drugs currently used in the treatment of IBS. Kaptchuk et al. (2008) concluded that factors contributing to the placebo effect can be progressively combined in a manner resembling a graded dose escalation of component parts and non-specific effects that can produce statistically and clinically significant outcomes. The patient–practitioner relationship is the most robust component (Kaptchuk et al., 2008).

A total of 638 adults with chronic mechanical low back pain were randomized to individualized acupuncture, standardized acupuncture, simulated acupuncture, or usual care. After 8 weeks of treatment, 60% of the patients who underwent placebo acupuncture (simulated acupuncture) and standardized acupuncture similarly manifested significant improvements of symptoms. On the other hand, only 39% of the patients receiving conventional treatments (usual care) manifested significant fewer improvements (Cherkin et al., 2009). They concluded that although acupuncture was found effective for chronic low back pain, tailoring needling sites to each patient and penetration of the skin appear to be unimportant in eliciting therapeutic benefits. It remains unclear whether acupuncture or simulated method of acupuncture provide physiologically important stimulation or represent placebo or nonspecific effects.

3.7.3. Acupuncturists' Behavior

The role of placebo effects elicited by acupuncturists' behavior has not been elucidated. Suarez-Almazor et al. (2010) recently reported the effects of acupuncturists' communication styles. Acupuncturists were trained to interact in 1 of 2 communication styles: high or neutral expectations. High expectations; acupuncturists conveyed high expectations of improvement, using positive utterances such as "I think this will work for you," "I've had a lot of success with treating knee pain," and "Most of my patients get better."

Neutral expectations; Acupuncturists conveyed uncertainty with utterances such as “It may or may not work for you,” “It really depends on the patient,” and “We’re uncertain, and that’s why we are doing the study,”

Statistically significant differences were observed in pain reduction and satisfaction, favoring the high expectations group. Acupuncturists' styles had significant effects on pain reduction and satisfaction, suggesting that the analgesic benefits of acupuncture can be partially mediated through placebo effects related to the acupuncturist's behavior (Suarez-Almazor et al., 2010).

3.7.4. Mental Activity of Expectation

Using a single blind, randomized crossover design with patients suffering from painful osteoarthritis, and PET scanning, Parient et al. (2005) studied the cerebral effects of needling and expectation on pain relief (non-specific therapeutic effect) with real acupuncture, placebo acupuncture (sham acupuncture) and skin pricks. The insula ipsilateral to the site of needling was activated to a greater extent during real acupuncture than during the placebo intervention. Real acupuncture and placebo (with the same expectation of effect as real acupuncture) cause greater activation than skin pricks (no expectation of a therapeutic effect) in the right dorsolateral prefrontal cortex (PFC), anterior cingulate cortex (ACC) and midbrain (Pariente et al., 2005).

As described in Chapter III, mental activity of expectation mediates placebo effects. The expectation initially activates PFC, resulting in the alteration of some other brain regions. These suggest that acupuncture has a specific physiological effect and that patients' expectation and belief regarding a potentially beneficial treatment modulate activity in component areas of the reward system

In general, most doctors have a negative feeling toward the placebo effects, because placebo effects are thought to be non-specific and/or psychological. However, it should be emphasized that emotional impact can alter brain activity, resulting in stimulation of various neurotransmitters and neuropeptides in the CNS. Placebo is a physiological mechanism as any other. Mental activity, conscious or unconscious, may modulate somatic mechanisms as effectively as any peripheral stimulus. When used together, somatic factors (real or sham acupuncture) and psychological factors (patient expectation and the acupuncturist-patient relationship) may act in harmony to provide the most effective use of endogenous mechanisms (Figure 4.7).

4. Transcutaneous Electrical Nerve Stimulation (TENS)

In contrast to acupuncture, transcutaneous electrical nerve stimulation (TENS) is a non-invasive procedure (Sluka et al., 2003), in which electrodes are placed on the skin and stimulated by electricity (Figure 4.8). It has been demonstrated that TENS, but not sham-TENS, showed a significant decrease of fMRI signal in the secondary somatosensory regions (Kara et al., 2010). TENS applied to the acupuncture points (transcutaneous-EA) at the hands and lower legs improved GI symptoms in patients with functional dyspepsia (FD) (Liu et al., 2008).

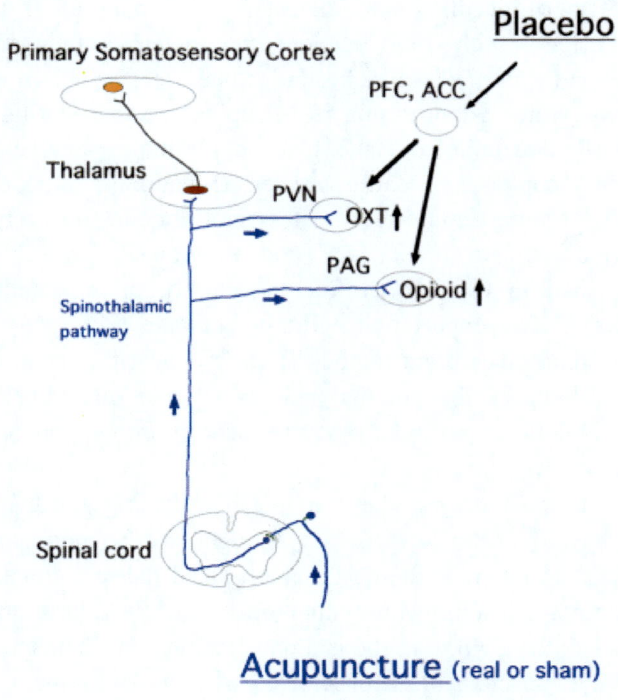

Figure 4.7. Psychological factors induced by expectation and acupuncturist-patient relationship (placebo effects) stimulate OXT and opioid release (black lines). The somatic factors stimulated by real or sham acupuncture also stimulate OXT and opioid release (blue lines). These two pathways act in harmony to utilize endogenous mechanisms most effectively.

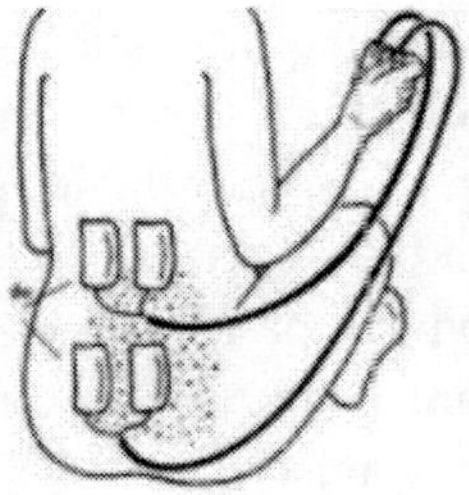

Figure 4.8. TENS.

TENS is a possible alternative candidate therapy for the treatment of patients suffering from stress-related diseases. TENS is side effect-free and cost-effective. TENS can be effectively done at home, is portable, requires little time commitment, and is easy to learn. TENS is a promising treatment for anxiety and/or GI disorders in any population of patients (Sallam et al., 2007).

Further clinical and basic studies are needed whether no needle insertion procedure (TENS) has similar effects on the somatosensory pathway, compared to the needle insertion procedure (acupuncture).

5. Massage Therapy

Massage therapy, the manual manipulation of soft tissue intended to promote health and well-being, has a history extending back several thousand years (Figure 4.9). Massage was a part of many ancient cultures including that of the Chinese, Egyptians, Greeks, Indians, Japanese, and Romans, and was often considered to be a medicinal practice.

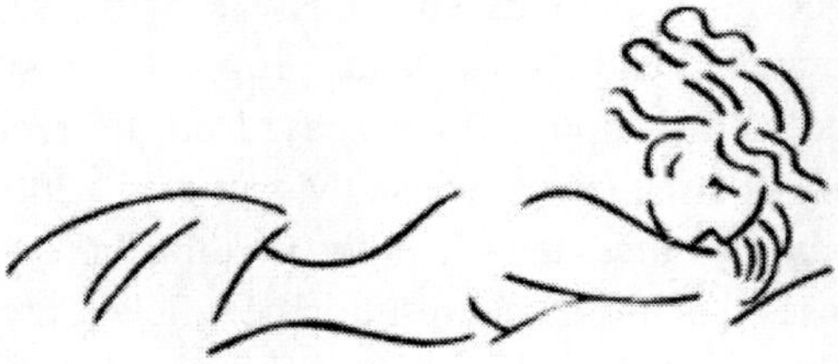

Figure 4.9. Massage.

Swedish massage is the most common form of massage in US, although it is not a pure form of therapy because most therapists integrate Swedish massage with other forms of touch therapy, such as acupressure. Swedish massage usually is given on a massage table, on the floor, or on a special massage chair and often with oil (vegetable or some aromatic oil). These oils are stroked and kneaded on all parts of the body. Smooth stroking and kneading-type movements are done up and down the back and across the shoulder muscles and the neck muscles and the backs of the legs, feet, arms, and hands. Stroking on the front is done across the stomach, the front of the legs and arms, and the face and forehead (Field, 2002).

The American massage therapy association (AMTA) defines massage as 'manual soft tissue manipulation that includes holding, causing movement, and/or applying pressure to the body,' and massage therapy as 'a profession in which the practitioner applies manual techniques, and may apply adjunctive therapies, with the intention of positively affecting the health and well-being of the client'.

Interest in massage therapy has continued to grow among the scientific community and consumers. Currently, massage therapy is one of the fastest growing sectors of the expanding CAM therapy movement in US. Visits to massage therapists increased 36% between 1990 and 1997, with consumers now spending $4-6 billion annually for massage therapy (Eisenberg et al., 1998), in pursuit of several benefits such as relaxation, feelings of well-being, and reductions in anxiety and pain (Moyer et al., 2004).

Massage therapy consists of a treatment lasting an hour or more, with firm strokes applied to numerous sites of the client's body in a private clinic. Clients also receive a 10-min treatment on the shoulders while seated in a public space such as a shopping mall or workplace.

Articles concerned with sports performance, exercise recovery, and injury management highlight the possibility that massage therapy may speed healing and reduce pain. The manipulations and pressure of massage therapy may break down subcutaneous adhesions and prevent fibrosis and promote circulation of blood and lymph, which may lead to reductions in pain associated with injury or strenuous exercise (Moyer et al., 2004). The pressure applied to the body by massage therapy is thought to trigger certain physiological responses that ultimately result in beneficial outcomes.

Twenty-eight adult patients with burns were randomly assigned to either a massage therapy group or a standard treatment control group. The behavior ratings of state, activity, vocalizations, and anxiety improved after the massage therapy sessions on the first and last days of treatment. Longer-term effects were also significantly better for the massage therapy group including decrease in depression and anger, and decreased pain (Field et al., 1998). Others showed that plasma cortisol level was decreased following massage therapy (Field et al., 1992; Ironson et al., 1996). Twenty-four women with premenstrual dysphoric disorder were randomly assigned to a massage therapy or a relaxation therapy group. The long term (5 week) effects of massage therapy included reduction in pain and water retention and overall menstrual distress (Hernandez-Reif et al., 2000). Soft tissue mobilization has been clinically successful in treating myofascial pain syndromes and other musculoskeletal dysfunctions. Soft tissue mobilization procedure elicited a somatovisceral-parasympathetic reflex. This suggests that massage therapy may increase parasympathetic tone and/or reduce excessive sympathetic activity (Cottingham et al., 1988).

Acupressure uses fingertips, rather than needles, to stimulate acupuncture points on the skin and has been implicated as a successful treatment for a variety of medical disorders. Acupressure treatment is effective in improving sleep quality in a sample of elderly residents at an assisted-living facility (Chen et al., 1999). Active acupressure reduced heart rate significantly more than did placebo acupressure (McFadden et al., 2010).

5.1. Mechanism of Beneficial Effects of Massage Therapy

5.1.1. Gate Control Theory

Melzack and Wall (1965) theorized that the experience of pain can be reduced by competing stimuli such as pressure or cold, because of the fact that these stimuli travel faster through nervous system pathways than pain (Gate control theory of pain reduction) (Melzack et al., 1965). Massage therapy performed with sufficient pressure would create a stimulus that interferes with the transmission of the pain stimuli to the brain, effectively "closing the gate" to the reception of pain before it can be processed (Barbour et al., 1986; Malkin, 1994; Field, 1998).

5.1.2. Autonomic Nervous System

Massage therapy may provide its benefits by shifting the autonomic nervous system from a state of sympathetic response to a state of parasympathetic response. The pressure applied during massage therapy may stimulate vagal activity (Field, 1998; Field, 2002), which in turn leads to a reduction of stress hormones and physiological arousal, and a subsequent parasympathetic response (Ferrell-Torry et al., 1993; Schachner et al., 1998; Hulme et al., 1999). Thus, massage therapy may promote reductions in anxiety, depression, and pain that are consistent with a state of calmness.

5.1.3. Stimulation of OXT System

OXT is associated with calmness, relaxed state, and positive emotions. Previous studies showed that OXT levels in plasma and cerebrospinal fluid (CSF) are increased in response to somatosensory nerve stimulation in humans (Stock et al., 1988; Uvnas-Moberg et al., 1993). In rats, high doses of OXT give rise to a sedative-like effect, including lowered blood pressure and reduced locomotion (Uvnas-Moberg, 1998a), while the physical stimulation of suckling itself produces anti-stress effects that include a lowered blood pressure and a decreased sympathetic tone (Uvnas-Moberg, 1996, 1998a).

There are many pieces of evidence, which shows that OXT is associated with physical touch. Human and animal studies suggested the anti-anxiety effect and anti-nociceptive effects of massage therapy are mediated via central release of OXT (Lund et al., 2002Bello, 2008 #2906; Rapaport et al., 2012).

In healthy young adults, the biologic effects of repeated Swedish massage therapy were compared to a light-touch control condition. The study comprised 45 minutes of Swedish massage or light touch, either weekly or twice weekly for 5 weeks. Compared to the touch control condition, weekly Swedish massage showed a minimal effect on HPA axis function. Twice-weekly massage produced a different response pattern with increased plasma OXT levels and decreased cortisol levels (Rapaport et al., 2012).

In rats, massage-like stroking of the abdomen raised plasma OXT levels with enhanced tolerance of pain (Agren et al., 1995). Similarly, repeated massage-like stroking resulted in increased OXT levels in plasma and PAG in rats. The long-term anti-nociceptive effects of massage-like stroking may be attributed to the OXTergic system (Lund et al., 2002).

It has been shown that stroking causes the relaxation with heart rate deceleration in dogs (Fonberg et al., 1981; Okamoto et al., 2009), suggesting that stroking might be good stimuli to inspire positive emotion. Once the abdominal area were stroked for 15 min, a significant rise of plasma OXT levels were observed in dogs (Mitsui et al., 2011)

It is occasionally suggested that some portion of massage therapy's effects may result from the interpersonal attention that the recipient experiences, as opposed to resulting entirely from the activation of physiological mechanisms. It is believed that interpersonal touch in the form of soft tissue manipulation is the sole reason that massage therapy groups show greater benefits than their comparison group.

As mentioned earlier, social grooming and or allogrooming play an important role in social bonding. Social support stimulates chronic OXT release, which has an anti-stress effect and also results in a long term reduction in blood pressure (Uvnas-Moberg, 1997b). OXT is involved with human attachment and contingent parenting in humans (Feldman et al., 2010). It is conceivable that a positive emotional interaction with the practitioner may stimulate the OXTergic system in the client. Thus, it is possible that both the psychological and physiological effects of massage therapy may be explained by OXT.

6. Spinal Manipulation (Chiropractic)

Manually applied movement and mobilization of body parts as a healing activity has been used for centuries. Spinal manipulation (chiropractic) is most commonly used by chiropractors, but other healthcare practitioners including osteopaths and physiotherapists also perform spinal manipulation. In spinal manipulation, a relatively high velocity and low amplitude force is applied to the vertebral column.

Spinal manipulation is believed to restore normal motion and normalize physiology of the neuro-musculoskeletal system in particular and potentially other physiological systems affected by the dysfunction. Spinal manipulation is typically applied when dysfunctional areas of the vertebral column are found. Clinicians identify these areas based upon changes in the texture and tone of paraspinal soft tissues, the ability to elicit pain and/or tenderness from these tissues, asymmetries in hard or soft tissue landmarks, and restrictions in spinal joint motion.

The concept of joint subluxation (a partial dislocation) in spinal manipulation proposes a biomechanical model of spinal pain that emphasizes normal function in the active, passive, and neural integration systems of the spine as a prerequisite for stability (Panjabi, 2006).

Meeker and Haldeman (2002) reviewed 43 randomized controlled trials using chiropractic for acute, subacute, and chronic low back pain. Thirty of these trials favored chiropractic over the comparison treatment. The remaining 13 reported no significant differences, and none reported that chiropractic was less effective than the comparison treatment (Meeker et al., 2002). Another analysis of systematic reviews including 69 trials concluded that spinal manipulation have a small to moderate benefits (Chou et al., 2007).

The mechanisms responsible for the therapeutic effects of spinal manipulation remain unclear. Spinal manipulation may produce a sustained change in the synaptic efficacy of central neurons by evoking a high frequency, bursting discharge from several types of dynamically sensitive, mechanosensitive paraspinal primary afferent neurons.

Pickar et al. (2012) proposed that spinal manipulation could affect the nervous system by activating paraspinal sensory neurons during the maneuver itself and/or by altering spinal biomechanics. Biomechanical changes which follow the manipulation would, in turn, modulate paravertebral sensory neuron signals (Pickar et al., 2012).

7. Music Therapy

Music is widely used to enhance well-being, reduce stress, and distract patients from unpleasant symptoms (Figure 4.10). Although there are wide variations in individual preferences, music appears to exert direct physiological effects through the autonomic nervous system. Music is a low-cost intervention that often reduces surgical, procedural, acute, and chronic pain. Music also improves the quality of life for patients receiving palliative care, enhancing a sense of comfort and relaxation (Kemper et al., 2005).

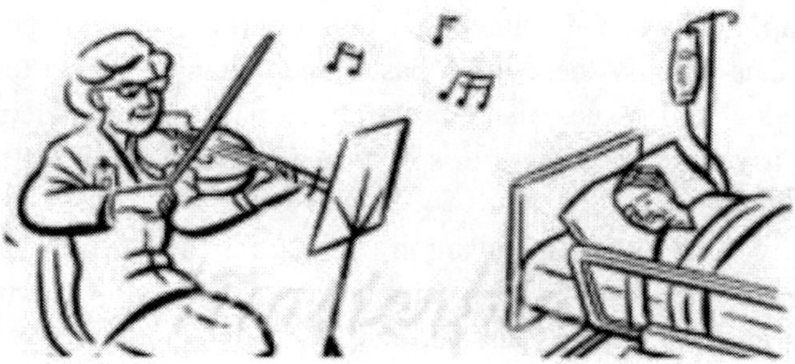

Figure 4.10. Music therapy.

It has been shown that music therapy can reduce anxiety and neurohormonal responses to psychological stress (Khalfa et al., 2003; Smith et al., 2004). Music therapy also reduces preoperative anxiety (Augustin et al.,

1996; Cooke et al., 2005) and postoperative pain (Nilsson et al., 2003; Voss et al., 2004; Nilsson et al., 2005). Some authors allowed patients to select the type of music (Augustin et al., 1996; Cooke et al., 2005), whereas others prefer to use new age (Voss et al., 2004; Nilsson et al., 2005) or classical music (Smith et al., 2004).

Sixty patients undergoing day surgery were randomized to one of three groups. Before and during surgery, patients in group-1 listened to new age music and those in group-2 listened to a choice of music from one of four styles. Patients in group-3 (control group) heard the normal sounds of the operating theatre. Plasma levels of cortisol were evaluated before, during and after operation. Plasma cortisol levels decreased during operation in both groups of patients who listened to music, but increased in the control group. Postoperative cortisol levels were significantly higher in group-1 than in group-2. These suggest that peri-operative music therapy changed the neurohormonal stress response to day surgery, especially when the type of music was selected by the patient (Leardi et al., 2007). The effectiveness of music therapy may depend on the type of music adopted in relation to the emotional perception of the patient.

The beneficial effect of singing on well-being was explored by Grape et al. (2003). It has been shown that OXT release is stimulated by pleasant sounds (Uvnas-Moberg, 1997b; Uvnas-Moberg et al., 2005; Dunbar, 2010).

Eight amateur and eight professional singers who had been attending singing lessons for at least six months were recruited. Plasma OXT concentrations increased significantly in both groups after the singing lesson. Amateurs reported increasing joy and elatedness, whereas professionals did not. However, both groups felt more energetic and relaxed after the singing lesson. The interviews showed that the professionals were clearly achievement-oriented, with focus on singing technique, vocal apparatus, and body during the lesson. The amateurs used the singing lessons as a means of self-actualization and self-expression to release emotional tension. Singing during a singing lesson seemed to promote more well-being and less arousal for amateurs compared to professional singers, who seemed to experience less well-being and more arousal (Grape et al., 2003).

In a randomized control study, patients undergoing cardiovascular surgery were exposed to two treatment arms: music listening and bed rest group and bed rest only group. The music and bed rest group exhibited higher levels of partial pressure of oxygen. The patients showed an increased relaxation associated with the higher plasma OXT levels (Nilsson, 2009). Thus, music listening is beneficial for cardiovascular system, may be due to increased OXT levels.

Music therapy may have anti-stress effects (Miluk-Kolasa et al., 1994; Fukui et al., 2003; Khalfa et al., 2003; Smith et al., 2004) and anti-nociceptive effects (Good et al., 1999; Renzi et al., 2000; Nilsson et al., 2003; Voss et al., 2004; Nilsson et al., 2005). As central OXT has anti-stress effects as well as anti-nociceptive effects, it is conceivable that beneficial effect of music therapy is mediated via increased OXT release.

Music also has indirect effects by modifying caregiver behavior. Providing music to caregivers may be a cost-effective and enjoyable strategy to improve empathy, compassion, and relationship-centered care while not increasing errors or interfering with technical aspects of care (Kemper et al., 2005).

8. Group Drumming

Group drumming is a recreational music making activity that builds social emotional assets consistent with a positive youth development approach (Figure 4.11). It is conducted in a circle and often led by a facilitator whose role is to maximize a sense of community through rhythmic dialogue. Group drumming is inclusive; it is non-verbal, universal, and does not require previous experience for participation. Furthermore, group drumming is culturally relevant; it is an integral part of diverse cultures, and supports the value of collectivism.

Previous studies have shown the bio-psycho-social efficacy of group drumming, using protocols involving reflection and self-disclosure to reduce stress (Bittman et al., 2001; Bittman et al., 2003; Bittman et al., 2004). These studies found neuroendocrine and immune changes that were indicative of reduced stress in normal adults with no previous experience in drumming (Bittman et al., 2001), reduced burnout and improved mood in long-term care workers and nurses (Bittman et al., 2003; Bittman et al., 2004), and improved social emotional functioning in adolescents.

The unique effectiveness of group drumming with reflection and self-disclosure, versus group drumming without these components, suggests the possible added benefit of integrating counseling activities with group drumming to reduce social and emotional manifestations of stress in low income youth (Bittman et al., 2001). Social–emotional skill building delivered in a framework of drumming may also confer benefits without the stigma of therapy.

Group drumming combined with group counseling activities would foster individual self-efficacy and positive outcome expectations through enactive attainment, vicarious experience, verbal persuasion and reduction of physiological arousal.

Low-income youth experience social-emotional problems linked to chronic stress that are exacerbated by lack of access to care. Low-income youth are in need of interventions to address social and emotional behavior linked to chronic stress. Therefore, a school-based group drumming program, integrated with activities from group counseling, can improve social and emotional behavior in low-income children.

Drumming is a non-verbal, universal activity that builds upon a collectivistic aspect of diverse cultures and does not bear the stigma of therapy. Participation in group drumming led to significant improvements in multiple domains of social-emotional behavior. This sustainable intervention can foster positive youth development and increase student-counselor interaction (Ho et al., 2011).

The beneficial effects of group drumming may be due to listening rhythmic music, exercise, and social interaction. The effects of exercise and social interaction on well-being are described Chapter V and VIII, respectively.

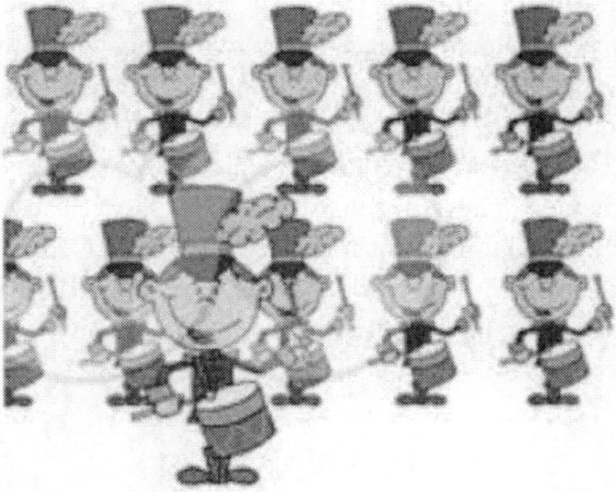

Figure 4.11. Group drumming.

9. Aromatherapy

Aromatherapy is a part of the discipline of phyto-therapy (the use of whole plants or parts of plants for medical purposes), and uses pure essential oils from fragrant plants (such as Peppermint, Sweet Marjoram, and Rose) to help relieve health problems and improve quality of life. Essential oils have been defined as non-oily, highly fragrant essences extracted from plants by distillation, which evaporate readily, and have been used by doctors in France for their antibiotic and antiviral properties for many years. They are most commonly used in oil burners, in bath water, or massaged into the skin, thus the aroma of the essential oil evaporates and stimulates the olfactory sense.

This is often then linked with a psychological response. Past experience may affect the subject's response in accordance with their like or dislike or the connotations of an aroma.

The emotional significance of an odor is provided by the role of the amygdala in the cerebral analysis of odor. Thus, there is increasing interest in any pharmacological action of aroma therapeutics. The healing properties of aromatherapy are claimed to include promotion of relaxation and sleep, relief of pain, and reduction of depressive symptoms, the rationale being that the essential oils have a calming and de-stressing effect. Aromatherapy might be of use as an intervention for people, who have little or no preserved language function. Aromatherapy has therefore been used for people with dementia to reduce disturbed behavior, and stimulate motivational behavior (Brooker et al., 1997; MacMahon et al., 1998).

Aromatherapy is frequently used in combination with other therapeutic approaches, such as massage. Aromatherapy is currently not under any licensing restrictions, and is easily accessible from pharmacies and health product stores. Therefore, there is a need for the effects of aroma therapy to be adequately documented (Thorgrimsen et al., 2003).

It has been shown that pleasant fragrance stimulates OXT release (Uvnas-Moberg, 1997b; Uvnas-Moberg et al., 2005; Dunbar, 2010), suggesting the mediation of OXT for the beneficial effects of aromatherapy.

Summary

Various types of manual therapies, such as acupuncture, TENS, and massage improve psychological disorders (anxiety and depression) and pain syndromes. Anti-stress effect of acupuncture is mediated via the stimulation of OXT release from the PVN (Figure 4.6). Anti-nociceptive effect and anti-emetic effect of acupuncture are mediated via the stimulation of opioid release from the PAG (Figure 4.7).

Placebo effects of acupuncture may involve somatic factors stimulated by real/sham acupuncture and psychological factors associated with expectation and acupuncturist-patient relationship (Figure 4.7). Beneficial effects of music therapy and aromatherapy may, at least in part, mediated via OXT release.

Chapter 5

PHYSICAL EXERCISE

Participation in physical exercise has been associated with the reduction of a number of physical (cardiovascular disease, colon and breast cancer, and obesity) and mental (depression and anxiety) disorders across the adult lifespan (Figure 5.1). Therefore, beneficial effects of physical exercise should be emphasized for the future medicine of integrative medicine.

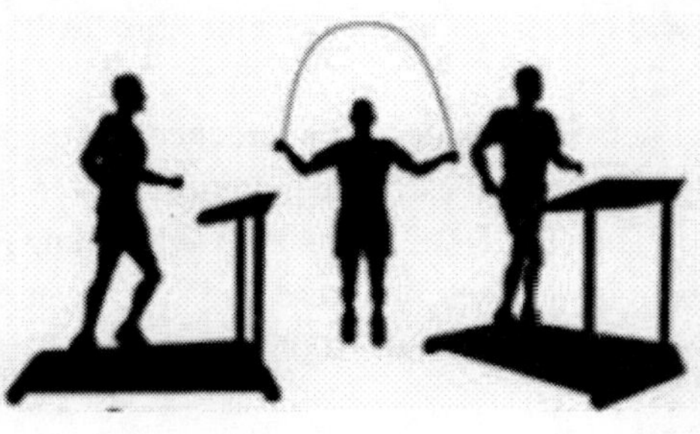

Figure 5.1.Physical Exercise.

Despite accumulated evidence for the importance of physical activity, 74% of adults in US do not meet the recommended guidelines of at least 30 minutes of moderate-intensity physical activity on most days (Hillman et al., 2008). Physical activity, as one the most important components of cardiovascular disease prevention, has crucial roles. Despite the strong evidence linking physical activity to cardiovascular disease risk reduction, there remains much uncertainty regarding the underlying mechanisms. In this

Chapter, the benefits of exercise are discussed as a modifiable life style parameter and its relation to our well-being.

Various types of physical exercises have shown possible physiological and psychological benefits. Psychological benefits include decreased depression, increased socialization and energy (Brugman et al., 2002), affective changes (Ekkekakis et al., 2000), and mood elevation (Lee et al., 2001b).

In addition, exercise training is beneficial for patients with hypertension (Higashi et al., 1999), diabetes (Maiorana et al., 2001), metabolic syndrome (Lavrencic et al., 2000), coronary artery disease (Gielen et al., 2003) and myocardial infarction (Vona et al., 2004), compared to those who do not participate in any training. Physical activity, such as aerobic exercise, has emerged as a promising low-cost treatment to improve neuro-cognitive function that is accessible to most adults and is not plagued by intolerable side effects often found with pharmaceutical treatments (Hillman et al., 2008).

The attitude toward exercise during and after cancer therapy has fundamentally changed over the years. Today, moderate physical activity is recommended instead of bed confinement at the beginning of cancer treatment. The undesired consequences of rest may include muscle atrophy and weakening of the immune system, whereas exercise not only reduces fatigue, depression, and anxiety but also enhances the health-related quality of life (Dobos et al., 2012).

Regular physical activity reduces the incidence of relapse and the risk of death by about 26%–40% in breast cancer patients after diagnosis. Patients with a body mass index (BMI) >25 are advised to engage in 5–7 hrs of moderate physical exercise a week, whereas 3–5 hrs a week are sufficient for patients with a BMI <25 (Holmes et al., 2005).

1. Anti-Stress Effects of Exercise

Stress is defined as a reaction to various real or perceived stimuli that threaten to disrupt the homeostatic state of the organism. Stress response is mediated by activation of hypothalamic-pituitary-adrenal (HPA) axis and the sympathetic nervous system, which results in increased secretion of cortisol and catecholamines, respectively. In the long-term over activation or dysregulation of the stress system may lead to the development of chronic disease.

Chronic psychosocial stress, in the presence of physical inactivity, is likely to contribute to the epidemic of cardiometabolic and emotional disease. On the other hand, regular exercise may prevent stress responses of daily life. Accumulating evidence documents the beneficial effects of regular exercise in preventing or ameliorating the metabolic and psychological comorbidities induced by chronic stress (Tsatsoulis et al., 2006). These benefits are thought to derive from the central effect of exercise to reduce the sensitivity to stress and also peripheral actions influencing metabolic functions.

1.1. Possible Mechanisms of Anti-Stress Effects

A randomized controlled trial examined the effect of physical exercise on depressive state, the excretion of stress hormones, and physiological fitness variables in adolescent females with mild depression. Twenty-four hour excretions of cortisol and epinephrine in urine were reduced by exercise regimen. The training group had a significantly reduced resting heart rate and increased peak oxygen uptake and lung capacity (Nabkasorn et al., 2006).

Exercise also stimulates the secretion of endogenous opioids and produces a state of euphoria (Grossman et al., 1984; Harber et al., 1984; Janal et al., 1984; Sher, 1998; Boecker et al., 2008). Exercise also promotes the secretion of neurotransmitters like serotonin and dopamine (Ransford, 1982).

1.1.1. Attenuation of HPA Axis

Forced swimming stress evoked a markedly enhanced response in cortisol levels in the exercising rats. In contrast, if rats were exposed to a novel environment, exercising rats showed much lower response in cortisol levels than the control animals. Thus, in exercising rats physically demanding stressors evoke enhanced cortisol responses whereas mild psychologically stressful stimuli such as novelty result in an attenuated cortisol response. The exercising rats showed less anxious behavior in the novelty situation. The changes in the sympatho-adrenomedullary input may play an important role in these distinct cortisol responses to stress (Droste et al., 2007).

1.1.2. Stimulation of Oxytocin (OXT) System

Receptors or nerve fibers are excited and shows rhythmic discharges by strong muscle contractions induced by protracted exercise. This somato-sensory stimulation induced by exercise may be carried to the brain stem and central nervous system (CNS), similarly to acupuncture stimulation (See

Chapter IV), resulting in the release of endogenous oxytocin (OXT) (Andersson et al., 1995). It has been shown that released OXT causes anti-stress effects via inhibiting corticotropin releasing factor (CRF) expression and HPA-axis (Bulbul et al., 2011).

2. ANTI-NOCICEPTIVE EFFECTS OF EXERCISE

The clinical benefits of exercise therapy for chronic pain are well established. Exercise is an effective treatment for various chronic musculoskeletal pain disorders, including chronic low back pain (van Middelkoop et al., 2010), chronic whiplash associated disorders (Stewart et al., 2007; Teasell et al., 2010) and osteoarthritis (Jansen et al., 2011).

In healthy individuals aerobic exercise of sufficient intensity activates pain inhibition for up to 30 minutes post-exercise (Koltyn, 2002). Anti-nociceptive effect of exercise is via the activation of central descending nociceptive inhibition in patients with osteoarthritis and rheumatoid arthritis (Van Oosterwijck et al., 2012).

In shoulder myalgia, exercising non-painful muscles activates generalized endogenous analgesia, but exercising painful muscles does not activate endogenous analgesia. Patients and healthy controls performed static contractions with quadriceps muscle (leg) and infraspinatus muscle (shoulder). Pressure pain thresholds increased at all sites during both contractions in healthy controls, but no increase was seen at any site during contractions in fibromyalgia patients, who even exhibited increased pain sensitivity. Myalgia patients had an increase in pressure pain thresholds at all sites during contraction of the non-painful quadriceps muscle, but no increase in pressure pain thresholds was seen at any site during contraction of the painful infraspinatus muscle. It was suggested, therefore, that nociceptive input from painful muscles induced central sensitization and activated descending pain facilitatory mechanisms. The facilitatory mechanisms could override the contraction-induced pain inhibition and explain the lack of generalized endogenous analgesia during contraction of painful muscles in myalgia patients and the increased pain sensitivity during contraction (Lannersten et al., 2010).

A dysfunctional response of some patients with chronic musculoskeletal pain to exercise has been shown. Several populations of chronic pain patients are unable to activate central descending nociceptive inhibition during exercise (Meeus et al., 2010; Van Oosterwijck et al., 2010; Van Oosterwijck et al.,

2012). Some chronic pain disorders (fibromyalgia and chronic fatigue syndrome) are characterized by a dysfunctional endogenous analgesia in response to both aerobic and local muscle exercises, while other chronic pain populations (chronic low back pain) show a normal activation of endogenous analgesia in response to exercise (Whiteside et al., 2004; Nijs et al., 2012).

2.1. Possible Mechanisms of Anti-Nociceptive Effects

2.1.1. Stimulation of Opioid and OXT System

Experimental and clinical studies suggest that afferent input in somatic nerve fibers has a significant effect on autonomic functions. As described in Chapter IV, acupuncture excites receptors or nerve fibers of the skin and muscles. Similarly, somatosensory neurons are also physiologically activated by strong muscle contractions induced by protracted exercise. Both exercise and acupuncture produce rhythmic discharges in nerve fibers, and cause the release of endogenous opioids and OXT. Endorphin levels have been observed to rise in the brain tissue of animals after both acupuncture and strong exercise (Uvnas-Moberg et al., 1993; Andersson et al., 1995).

The exercise-induced analgesia is presumably due to the release of endogenous opioids from the PAG (Koltyn et al., 1998; Koltyn, 2000) and OXT from the hypothalamus (Breton et al., 2009; Rojas-Piloni et al., 2010), which activates supra-spinal nociceptive inhibitory mechanisms (Millan, 2002; Ray et al., 2007). It is likely that exercise therapy may induce desensitization of CNS.

These mechanisms might be related to cardiovascular changes (increase in heart rate and blood pressure) during exercise (Koltyn et al., 2006). The exercise-induced blood pressure increase activates arterial baro-receptors, resulting in increased supraspinal inhibition (Ghione, 1996; Koltyn et al., 2006)) and stimulation of brain centers involved in pain modulation (Dworkin et al., 1994).

2.1.2. Stimulation of Serotonergic (5-HT) Neurons

Serotonergic (5-HT) neurons are implicated in modulating nociceptive transmission. It has been demonstrated that 5-HT neuronal activity is enhanced by rhythmic behaviors such as chewing and locomotion in animals (Jacobs et al., 1993). Mohri et al. (2005) showed that 5-HT descending inhibitory pathways are enhanced by rhythmic behavior of gum chewing in humans. Serotonin transporters have recently been discovered at the blood-brain barrier

(BBB), suggesting that the rise in blood 5-HT may possibly reflect an increase in 5-HT level within the brain. Thus, the rhythmic behaviors may suppress nociceptive responses via the 5-HT descending inhibitory pathway (Mohri et al., 2005).

3. Cardiovascular Effects of Exercise

The American Heart Association recommends at least 30 minutes of moderate (at 50–70% of maximal predicted heart rate) exercise on most days to reduce the risk of cardiovascular events. Human studies demonstrated that chronic aerobic exercise regimens improve cardiovascular function in older people (Benjamin et al., 2004) and those with cardiovascular risk factors (Hambrecht et al., 1998), as well as healthy young subjects (Clarkson et al., 1999).

Regular physical exercise corrected the endothelial dysfunction of the skeletal muscle vasculature and improved exercise capacity in patients with chronic heart failure (Hambrecht et al., 1998). In patients with stable coronary artery disease, exercise training showed an improved endothelium-dependent vasodilatory capacity (Hambrecht et al., 2003). Ten-week, aerobic and anaerobic exercise training enhanced endothelium-dependent dilation in healthy young men. This may contribute to the benefit of regular exercise in preventing cardiovascular disease (Clarkson et al., 1999).

3.1. Possible Mechanisms of Improved Cardiovascular Function

3.1.1. Free Radicals

Free radicals are physiological byproducts of aerobic metabolism and are widely recognized for their dual roles as both deleterious and beneficial species, since they can be either harmful or beneficial to living systems (Valko et al., 2006). High concentrations of free radicals harm living organisms through reactions with adjacent molecules (proteins, lipids, carbohydrates, and nucleic acids). As a result, mammalian cells have evolved a variety of antioxidant mechanisms to control free radicals production and propagation (Fridovich, 1999). On the other hand, mild oxidative stress can act as a stimulant of physiological antioxidant systems and as a trigger for various physiological adaptations (Gomez-Cabrera et al., 2008).

3.1.2. Endothelial Nitric Oxide Synthase (eNOS)

The vascular endothelium plays a vital role in regulating arterial dilation by manufacturing vasodilator (nitric oxide; NO). A key component of intact endothelial function is NO production by endothelial nitric oxide synthase (eNOS). The anti-inflammatory, vasodilatory and platelet inhibitory effect of NO have important roles in the maintenance of vascular hemostasis (Vita, 2002). The risk of cardiovascular events such as myocardial infarction or ischemic stroke was 3-4 folds higher in cardiovascular patients with endothelial dysfunction compared to those with a normal endothelial function (Lerman et al., 2005).

Physical activity increases vascular expression of eNOS in mice (Fukai et al., 2000) and humans (Hambrecht et al., 2003). Exercise-induced up-regulation of vascular eNOS expression is closely related to the changes of frequency and the intensity of physical forces within the vasculature, especially shear stress. Exercise induced increase in heart rate may enhance cardiac output and vascular shear stress, leading to increased expression of eNOS (Fleming et al., 2003; Golbidi et al., 2012).

3.1.3. Autonomic Nervous System

It is well known that cardiac output, total peripheral resistance, and venous capacitance are neurally regulated to keep blood pressure and volume, maintaining adequate blood supply to different vasculatures. To maintain blood pressure and efficiently adjust flow to several territories in different environmental situations, the CNS processes peripheral information conveyed by different sets of receptors such as baro-receptors and chemo-receptors. The peripheral information is integrated in different areas and at different levels of the CNS to provide adequate changes in sympathetic and parasympathetic tone to the heart and blood vessels (Potts, 2001).

The nucleus tractus solitarius (NTS) neurons of the brain stem receive synaptic input from many sensory modalities. It has been shown that neurons in the NTS are the primary targets for somatic afferent fibers activated by skeletal muscle contraction. Local inhibition of baroreceptor signaling is necessary to counteract the increase in baroreceptor input such that NTS output is normalized and baro-reflex sensitivity is maintained during exercise (Potts, 2001). The activation of ascending spinal neurons from the cervical dorsal horn by contraction-sensitive skeletal muscle afferents selectively inhibits arterial baroreceptor signaling in the NTS (Potts et al., 2003).

4. Improved Memory Function by Exercise

An emerging body of multidisciplinary literature has documented the beneficial influence of physical activity engendered through aerobic exercise on selective aspects of brain function. Human and animal studies have shown that aerobic exercise can improve a number of aspects of cognition and performance. It is true that exercise can help to improve the academic performance as well as physical health.

Animal research has shown that enriched environments, including access to exercise equipment (such as running wheels), has a positive effect on neuronal growth and on the neural systems that are involved in learning and memory (Vaynman et al., 2006). Exercise enhances learning and improves retention, which is accompanied by increased cell proliferation and survival in the hippocampus in aged mice (van Praag et al., 2005). In human research by neuro imaging techniques, exercise leads to evident changes in brain structure and function (Booth et al., 2006).

4.1. Possible Mechanism of Improved Brain Function

Brain derived neurotrophic factor (BDNF) system plays a critical role in interface metabolism and cognition. BDNF is a neurotrophin, a regulator of the survival, growth, and differentiation of neurons during development (Barde, 1994; Wang et al., 1995). BDNF functions to translate activity into synaptic and cognitive plasticity in the adult animal. BDNF is able to modulate the efficacy of neurotransmitter release (Bolton et al., 2000), and stimulate the synthesis of vesicle-associated proteins (Lu et al., 1999).

Human studies support the importance of BDNF in learning and memory (Egan et al., 2003; Hariri et al., 2003). Learning, memory and long-term potentiation (LTP) selectively increase BDNF mRNA levels in the hippocampus (Falkenberg et al., 1992). The hippocampus shrinks in late adulthood, leading to impaired memory and increased risk for dementia. Hippocampal and medial temporal lobe volumes are larger in higher-fit adults, and physical activity training increases hippocampal perfusion. In a randomized controlled trial with 120 older adults, aerobic exercise training increased the size of the anterior hippocampus, leading to improvements in spatial memory. Exercise training increased hippocampal volume by 2%, effectively reversing age-related loss in volume.

Increased hippocampal volume is associated with greater serum levels of BDNF. Hippocampal volume declined in the control group, but higher pre-intervention fitness partially attenuated the decline, suggesting that fitness protects against volume loss. These suggest that aerobic exercise training is effective at reversing hippocampal volume loss in late adulthood, which is accompanied by improved memory function (Erickson et al., 2011).

5. Beneficial Effects of Group Exercise

Exercise environments providing opportunities for social interaction result in enhanced affect (McAuley et al., 2000a; McAuley et al., 2000b). This may be related to experiences of social inclusion through friendship and feeling like a worthwhile human being through meaningful activity. Davidson et al. (2001) explain how social interaction helps people to relax, unwin and distract themselves from their ongoing suffering (Davidson et al., 2001a; Davidson et al., 2001b).

The beneficial effects of group exercise may be due to social interaction. It has been shown that hypothalamic OXT is activated in response to social interaction. OXT is linked to health-promoting cardiovascular, analgesic, anti-inflammatory and anti-stress effects (See Chapter VII).

Summary

Various types of physical exercises have shown possible physiological and psychological benefits. Anti-stress effect of exercise is mediated via the reduction of HPA axis. Anti-nociceptive effect of exercise is mediated via the release of opioid from the PAG and OXT from the hypothalamus. Physical exercise delays the accumulation of free radical-mediated cell damage, increases eNOS expression and alters autonomic nerve function. These may lead to improved cardiovascular function.

Chapter 6

HERBS

The use of herbal medicine began in ancient China at the time of Xia dynasty and in India during the Vedic period (Figure 6.1). In the last 2-3 decades, the use of herbal medicine in the form of complementary and alternative medicine (CAM) has been popular in the Western countries. There has been a five-fold increase in the use of herbal medicines within the last decade. In US, adults use herbal products with gross sales surpassing $5 billion annually (Eisenberg et al., 1998). It is estimated that at least 20% of adult Americans taking prescription medications also use herbal products, megavitamins, or both. It should be noted that many individuals did not receive any advice from CAM practitioners. They frequently made the choice of their own, just by perusing products on a shelf at the local nutrition store (Leak, 1999).

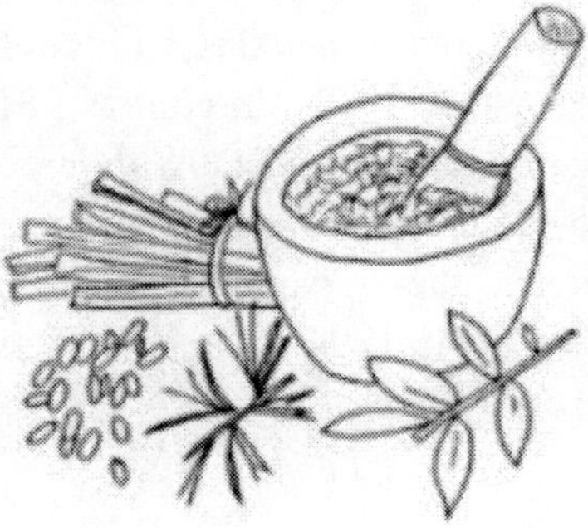

Figure 6.1. Herbs.

1. Efficacy

Herbal medicines are gaining importance and expanding throughout the world, mainly due to easy availability, natural way of healing, and less side effects. The widespread use of herbs is emphasized among people with chronic disease, since it helps to avoid dissatisfaction often associated with conventional health care (Astin, 1998). Herbs are believed to be safer and better than standard medical practice because they are natural. Treatments with herbal medicine concentrate on re-establishing or reinforcing natural healing processes and wellness. While there are many herbal products available, garlic, ginkgo, ginseng, and ginger have been favored in the US.

1.1. Garlic

Historically, garlic (*Allium sativum*) has been used for colds, sore throats, intestinal disorders, rheumatism, and coughs as well as a diuretic. Garlic is reported to be the third most popular herbal supplement in US, with sales exceeding $19 million per year. It is used raw as a seasoning or condiment, and as an extract in dietary supplements. Fresh garlic and garlic in dietary supplement form may have different physiological effects and properties, with both forms purported to have anti-bacterial and cholesterol-lowering properties (Stanger et al., 2011).

Meta-analysis of the controlled trials of garlic to reduce hypercholesterolemia showed a significant reduction in total cholesterol levels. The best available evidence suggests that garlic, in an amount approximating one half to one clove per day, decreased total serum cholesterol levels by about 9% in the groups of patients in persons with cholesterol levels greater than 200 mg/dl (Warshafsky et al., 1993). In contrast, Silagy and Neil (1994) performed a meta-analysis on eight studies with a total of 415 patients. Although there was some evidence of anti-hypertensive effect, due to less than adequate testing parameters, there was little to suggest on absolute cardiovascular benefit (Silagy et al., 1994).

1.2. Ginkgo

Ginkgo (*Ginkgo biloba*) is among the top ten best-selling herbs in US, with sales exceeding $17 million per year. Several manufacturers have added ginkgo to their multi-vitamin and other multi-component products in amounts that vary from 40 mg to 240 mg/day. Gingko can also be found in energy drinks in varying amounts (Stanger et al., 2011). Ginkgo is frequently used for circulatory stimulant, tinnitus, vertigo and enhancement of memory. It has been proposed that ginkgo's effects on platelet activating factor inhibition may enhance its anti-inflammatory effect (Braquet et al., 1987). Ginkgo acts as a free radical scavenger, and that it affects platelet activating factor inhibition, both of which have beneficial effects on vasculature (Leak, 1999).

Because of its strong anti-oxidant qualities, ginkgo may have great use in treating Alzheimer's disease. In their double blind, placebo-controlled multi-center study, LeBars et al. (1997) found those patients with multi-infarct dementia and Alzheimer's disease had improvement, or at least no worsening in their socialization and cognitive skills (Le Bars et al., 1997). However, it seems less possibility of a preventive effect in healthy persons. In a 42-month pilot study with cognitively intact subjects ginkgo neither altered the risk of progression from normal to clinical dementia, nor protected against a decline in memory function (Dodge et al., 2008). In volunteers above 74 years with normal cognition or mild cognitive impairment at study entry, ginkgo at 240 mg/day for a median of 6 years did not reduce the incidence rate of dementia and Alzheimer's (DeKosky et al., 2008).

1.3. Ginseng

Ginseng (*Panax ginseng*) is a perennial herb found in Korea and China. It has been used in eastern Asian herbal remedies for thousands of years as a stimulant and aphrodisiac and is presently marketed in US and many other countries to increase alertness and energy. Ginseng was used in ancient times for long life, vigor, and strength. Globally, sales of ginseng exceeded $ 1.5 billion in 2008 (Stanger et al., 2011).

In a double-blind study done in 1982 on night duty nursing performance, Hallstrom (1982), found that nurses on ginseng had an improved sense of well- being and were more competent (Hallstrom, 1982). However, another double-blind, placebo controlled clinical study showed less benefit of ginseng for quality of life and psychomotor performance in healthy volunteers (Wiklund et al., 1986).

1.4. Ginger

Ginger is the rhizome of the plant *Zingeber officinale*. Ginger is one of the classic examples of an herb used for not only culinary preparations but also for unique therapeutic significance owing to its anti-oxidant, anti-microbial, and anti-inflammatory properties. The pungent fractions of ginger (*gingerols, shogaols, and paradols*) are mainly attributed to the health-enhancing perspectives of ginger (Butt et al., 2012). Medicinally, it has been used to alleviate nausea (Lien et al., 2003). The recommended daily dose of ginger is 1 g daily. Amounts exceeding 4 g may cause stomach discomfort and nausea. Ginger has also been reported to lower cholesterol levels and to have blood-thinning properties (Verma et al., 1993).

2. Interaction between Herbs and Drugs

Almost 60% of patients fail to disclose alternative therapy use (including herbals) to their physicians (Eisenberg et al., 1998). Moreover, physicians used to focus attention on potential toxicities, even though identification of toxicity from herbal preparations is often difficult, because patients generally self medicate with these and may withhold this information.

As the use of complementary medicine grows, it is likely that concurrent use of herbs with drugs may mimic, magnify, or oppose the effect of drugs leading to herb-drug interactions. Health-care practitioners should caution patients against mixing herbs and pharmaceutical drugs. However, there is very little information published on herb-herb or herb-drug interactions as compared to the use of herbs.

Hermann and Richter (2012) recently provided summaries of clinical herb-drug interaction (Hermann et al., 2012). Common herbal medicines that interact with drugs include St John's wort, ginkgo, ginger, ginseng, and garlic. The common drugs that interact with herbal medicines include warfarin, midazolam, digoxin, amitriptyline, indinavir, cyclosporine, tacrolimus and irinotecan. Herbal medicines may interact with drugs at the intestine, liver, kidneys, and targets of action (Chen et al., 2012b).

Cytochrome P450 (CYP) inhibition or induction is probably the most common mechanism for the pharmacokinetic interactions of herbs and drugs. Any inhibition of CYP enzymes by herbal extracts may result in enhanced plasma and tissue concentration of drugs, leading to toxicity, while induction results in reduced drug concentration leading to decreased drug efficacy and treatment failure (Mukherjee et al., 2011).

3. Adverse Effects

Despite increasing popularity, communication about the use of herbs between physicians and patients is limited: most physicians know little about herbs and patients avoid discussing CAM because they fear being received with indifference (Deng et al., 2007). Up to 15 million users may be at risk for potential adverse interactions between these alternative products or their prescriptions.

Unlike conventional medicines, herbal remedies are not regulated by governmental agencies such as FDA. The Dietary and Supplement Health and Education Act of 1994 classified herbal remedies as dietary supplements, which rendered them exempt from the safety and efficacy regulations required of prescription and over-the-counter medications. Recent review article provided the adverse effects of herbal remedies including the most widely sold herbal medicinal products and reinforce the safety aspect of herbal products, (Singh et al., 2011).

It has been suggested that some herbs could adversely affect coagulation when taken alone or in combination with anti-platelet medications. Herbs could alter hemostasis by a variety of mechanisms, such as reducing platelet aggregation or inhibiting arachidonic acid, a cellular signaling messenger and inflammatory intermediate. Moderate to severe adverse events, such as spinal epidural hematoma, spontaneous intracerebral hemorrhage, retrobulbar hemorrhage, and subarachnoid hemorrhage have occasionally been anecdotally associated with consumption of herbs (Stanger et al., 2011).

Summary

Although the use of herbal medicine has been popular in the Western countries, many individuals did not receive any advice from CAM practitioners. Because of the possible herb-drug interactions, health-care practitioners should caution patients against mixing herbs and pharmaceutical drugs. Some herbs could adversely affect coagulation when taken alone or in combination with anti-platelet medications.

Chapter 7

ROLE OF OXYTOCIN IN WELL-BEING

The beneficial effects of manual therapies (acupuncture and massage), music therapy, and meditation are, at least in part, mediated via oxytocin (OXT) release in the brain. OXT also plays an important role in placebo effects and doctor-patient relationships. Thus, the physiological role of central OXT has a strong association with the concept of integrative medicine.

OXT exerts a wide spectrum of central and peripheral effects as a neurohormone, neurotransmitter, or neuromodulator. In the central nervous system (CNS), OXT is produced in the neurons of the supraoptic nuclei (SON) and paraventricular nuclei (PVN) of the hypothalamus (Figure 7.1) and is mainly released from the neurohypophysis (posterior pituitary gland) and nerve terminals in response to multiple physiological stimuli (Cazalis et al., 1987b, a; Nordmann et al., 1988).

Besides its well-known physiological functions such as uterus contraction and milk ejection, OXT plays an important role in regulating social behavior and positive social interactions (Neumann, 2008). The recent researches indicate that OXT plays an important role in mother-infant bonding, social attachment, trust, self-healing, and mind-body connection (Carter, 1992; Uvnas-Moberg, 1996). OXT is also linked to health-promoting cardiovascular, metabolic, analgesic, anti-inflammatory and anti-stress effects (Babygirija et al., 2010; Gutkowska et al., 2012).

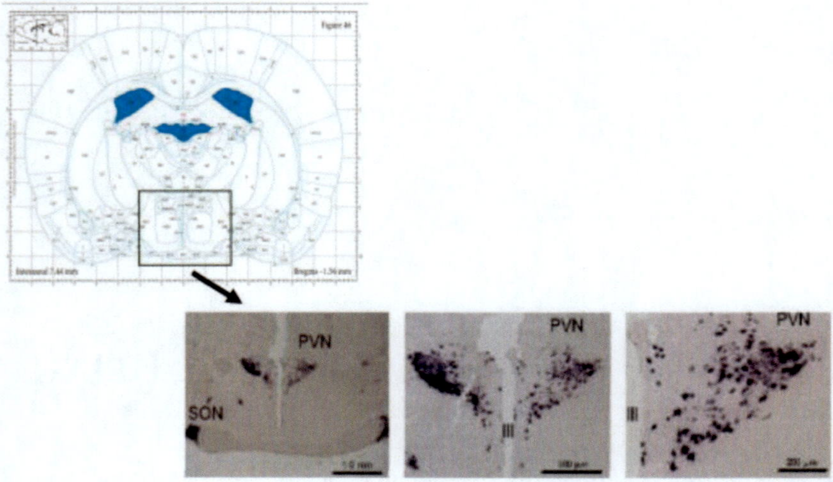

Figure 7.1. Oxytocin producing neurons at the hypothalamus (PVN and SON).

It has been suggested that the increase in OXT is related to calmness and relaxed state (Miller, 2009). Human and animal studies have shown that OXT system is stimulated by various stimuli, such as sight (Strathearn et al., 2009), touch (Grewen et al., 20051; Bello et al., 2008), smell (Hernandez et al., 2002), food intake (Verbalis et al., 1986), exercise (Michelini et al., 2001), and social attachment (Carter, 1998; Uvnas-Moberg et al., 2005).

1. Social Attachment

As humans are social creatures, prosocial behavior is critical for the individual to interact with the environment. Impairment in social behavior is associated with decreased quality of life and psychopathological states (Heinrichs et al., 2003). Access to a supportive network reduced the risk of cardiovascular disease. The social support stimulates chronic OXT release, resulting in long term reduction in blood pressure and anti-stress effects through mediating secondary effects (Uvnas-Moberg, 1997b).

In various animal models, OXT has been shown to increase social contact between individuals and thereby facilitating bonding or attachment (Carter, 1992; Uvnas-Moberg, 1996; Babygirija et al., 2010). Centrally infused OXT enhances adult social interactions in male rats (Witt et al., 1992). Mice mutant for the OXT gene (OXT knockout mice; OXT-KO mice) fails to develop social recognition, whereas wild type mice (normal mice) show intact social recognition. Treatment with OXT rescues social recognition in OXT-KO mice, while treatment with an OXT antagonist produced a social amnesia-like effect in wild type mice (Ferguson et al., 2000).

Paired housing has been shown to reduce the long-term adverse behavioral and physiological effects of social defeat on cardiovascular, neuroendocrine and behavioral responses in rats (Ruis et al., 1999; Sharp et al., 2002). Paired housing facilitates wound healing via attenuating the activity of HPA axis in male monogamous mice (Glasper et al., 2005). Increased activity of OXT during mating is directly linked to an attenuated anxiety-related behavior in male rats (Neumann, 2008). Thus, it is highly likely that social interactions induced by paired housing upregulate hypothalamic OXT expression resulting in attenuation of HPA axis.

Socially isolated mice with nerve injury developed depressive-like behavior, which was attenuated by the central administration of OXT. Conversely, pair-housed animals treated with OXT receptor antagonist developed depressive-like behavior (Norman et al., 2010). These suggest that social interaction alters the affective responses to nerve injury through a mechanism involving OXTergic system.

Plasma OXT and salivary OXT in mothers' and fathers' were associated with parent and child's social engagement, affected synchrony, and positive communicative sequences between parent and child. Plasma OXT and salivary OXT were associated with mothers' and fathers' attachment relationships throughout life. These suggest that OXT is involved in human attachment and contingent parenting in humans (Feldman et al., 2010).

Couples who received OXT before the standardized couple conflict discussion had significantly reduced anxiety levels, as indicated by subjective evaluation and reduced salivary cortisol levels. The OXT group also showed increased positive communication behavior and less negative behavior during the conflict session (Ditzen et al., 2009).

Hypothalamic-pituitary-adrenal (HPA) axis plays a major role in initiating stress-responses, and hypothalamic OXT reduces the activity of HPA axis. There was a recurrent association between high levels of activity in the HPA axis and the subsequent expression of social behaviors and attachments. Positive social behavior reduces HPA axis activity, while negative social interactions can have the opposite effect. Social interactions and attachment involve endocrine systems capable of attenuating HPA axis activity and modulating the autonomic nervous system (Carter, 1998).

2. Trust

Trust is indispensable in friendship, love, families and organizations, and plays a key role in economic exchange and politics. Human beings exhibit substantial interpersonal trust even with strangers. Plasma OXT levels are higher in subjects who received a monetary transfer that reflects an intention of trust relative to an unintentional monetary transfer of the same amount. In addition, higher OXT levels are associated with trustworthy behavior (the reciprocation of trust). It is suggested that perceptions of intentions of trust affect levels of circulating OXT (Zak et al., 2005).

The blood brain barrier (BBB) is the separation of circulating blood from the brain extracellular fluid in the central nervous system (CNS). As OXT is a relatively large hydrophilic molecule, it is generally accepted that OXT does not cross BBB, indicating that peripherally administered OXT may not affect brain function. There is abundant indirect evidence for the "nose to brain" pathway as determined by the efficacy of intranasally administered OXT in clinical trials. Intranasal administration of OXT spray promotes a substantial increase in trusting behavior. Intranasal administration of OXT specifically affects an individual's willingness to accept social risks arising through interpersonal interactions. OXT causes a substantial increase in trust among humans, thereby greatly increasing the benefits from social interactions (Kosfeld et al., 2005). These results suggest the essential role for OXT in the development of trusting behavior.

Baumgartner et al. (2008) examined the neural circuitry of trusting behavior by combining the intranasal, double blind administration of OXT with functional magnetic resonance imaging (fMRI). The subjects in the OXT administration group showed no change in their trusting behavior after they learned that their trust had been breached several times, while subjects receiving placebo decrease their trust. This difference in trust adaptation is associated with a specific reduction in activation in the amygdala, the midbrain regions, and the dorsal striatum in subjects receiving OXT. This suggests that neural systems mediating fear processing (amygdala and midbrain regions) and behavioral adaptations to feedback information (dorsal striatum) modulate effects of OXT on trust (Baumgartner et al., 2008).

3. ANTI-STRESS EFFECTS OF OXT

Stress affects mind, body, and behavior in many ways, and everyone experiences stress differently. Social contact has been shown to play an integral role in psychological and physiological well-being for several species. When animals are subjected to stress, corticotropin releasing factor (CRF) is secreted from the hypothalamus, which results in the secretion of corticosterone (cortisol) from the adrenal cortex to guard against stress disorders.

In response to psychological stressors, there is a dose dependent effect of OXT in attenuating stress-induced HPA activation on neural circuits including the PVN. OXT administration significantly attenuated the release of ACTH and cortisol and the increase in CRF mRNA expression in the PVN in response to acute restraint stress (Windle et al., 2004). Acute or chronic central administration of OXT reduces stress responses in rats (Windle et al., 1997) and mice (Ring et al., 2006).

OXT induces a subjective feeling of general well-being through suppression of anxiety, hostility and fear (Uvnas-Moberg, 1997a, 1998b). In human studies, the intranasal OXT administration exhibited increased calmness and decreased anxiety in response to the social stress loading. The anxiolytic (anti-anxiety) effect was greatest in those who had both social support and OXT administration (Heinrichs et al., 2003). Thus, OXT seems to enhance the buffering effect of social support on stress responsiveness.

For anxiety disorders, patients are often given supportive medications such as selective serotonin reuptake inhibitors (SSRIs) and diazepam (a minor tranquilizer). One of the actions of SSRIs is through increased OXT release (Uvnas-Moberg, 1996; Uvnas-Moberg et al., 1999). Administration of SSRIs increased plasma OXT levels in rats (Uvnas-Moberg et al., 1999). The median raphe nucleus is a main site of action for SSRI anti-depressants. OXT infusion facilitated serotonin (5-HT) release within the median raphe nucleus and reduces anxiety-related behavior in mice. Infusion of a 5-HT receptor antagonist blocks the anxiolytic effect of OXT, suggesting that OXT receptor activation in 5-HT neurons mediates the anxiolytic effects of OXT. Thus, OXT may regulate 5-HT release and exert anxiolytic effects via direct activation of OXT receptor expressed in 5-HT neurons of the raphe nuclei (Yoshida et al., 2009).

Stress is widely believed to play a major role in the development of functional gastrointestinal (GI) disorders. Patients with serious stress frequently complain of GI symptoms and these symptoms are, at least in part, likely due to GI dysmotility (abnormal GI motility). Gastric emptying was delayed and colonic transit was accelerated following chronic stress loading in rats. Central-administration of OXT significantly improved the dysmotility of GI tract (Zheng et al., 2010; Yoshimoto et al., 2012b). Patients with functional GI disorders often report symptoms that are more associated with negative life changes. Social attachment is likely to overcome the daily stressful events and improve GI dysmotility via up-regulating central OXT expression (Babygirija et al., 2010).

3.1. Mechanism of Anti-Stress Effects of OXT

The inhibitory effect of OXT may not directly act on CRF neurons, because the majority of neuronal responses to OXT are excitatory (Inenaga et al., 1986). Gamma-aminobutyric acid (GABA) is the major inhibitory amino acid transmitter of the mammalian CNS. GABAergic neurons are located in the immediate surroundings of the PVN (peri-PVN), especially at the dorsal part of the PVN (Roland et al., 1993). These GABA-projecting neurons into the PVN are known to inhibit CRF expression via $GABA_A$ receptors (Bali et al., 2003; Cullinan et al., 2008).

GABA exerts its effects through $GABA_A$ and $GABA_B$ receptors (Kuffler et al., 1958; Krnjevic et al., 1967; Curtis et al., 1970). $GABA_A$ receptors are expressed on the CRF neurons at the PVN (Cullinan, 2000). Released corticosterone in response to acute stress inhibits CRF release via a feedback mechanism, which is mediated via $GABA_A$ receptors in the PVN (Di et al., 2008). A recent animal study suggests that OXT inhibits stress-induced CRF expression via $GABA_A$ receptors in the PVN (Bulbul et al., 2011) (Figure 7.2).

The anxiolytic agent, diazepam, is a $GABA_A$ receptor agonist (a stimulant of $GABA_A$ receptor). Interestingly, animal studies showed that subcutaneous administration of low dose of OXT has an anxiolytic effect very similar to clinically used diazepam (Uvnas-Moberg et al., 1994). It is likely that the anxiolytic affect of OXT is mediated via $GABA_A$ receptors at the PVN.

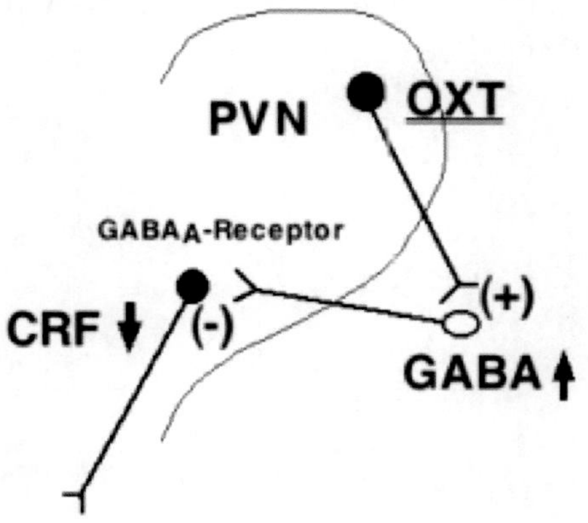

Figure 7.2. OXT inhibits stress-induced CRF mRNA expression via $GABA_A$ receptors in the PVN.

4. Anti-Nociceptive Effects

In addition to opioid system, recent studies suggested that anti-nociceptive effect of somatosensory stimulation is mediated via OXT system itself (Stock et al., 1988; Uvnas-Moberg et al., 1993; Agren et al., 1995; Yang et al., 2007). Greater OXT levels were correlated with greater tolerance to ischemic pain or cold pressor pain in healthy women. Reduced OXTergic function may be one of multiple biological factors contributing to the greater sensitivity to experimental ischemic pain (Grewen et al., 2008).

The descending inhibitory system also receives a wide array of afferent modulations from the supra-brainstem regions, including hypothalamus. It has been documented that there is direct descending OXT neuron projection from the PVN to the spinal cord. This is the way by which stimulation of hypothalamic OXT neurons modulates nociceptive responses (Breton et al., 2009; Rojas-Piloni et al., 2010).

The possible mechanisms of anti-nociceptive effects of hypothalamic OXT are; (1) a direct descending projection of OXTergic neurons from the PVN to spinal cord and modulation of spinal dorsal horn neurons (#1; spinal pathway); (2) a descending projection of OXTergic neurons from the PVN to PAG to enhance opioid release (#2; ponto-medullary pathway); (**3**) OXT-induced inhibition on CRF release and reduction of systemic cortisol (#3; CRF-HPA axis pathway) (Figure 7.3). Clinical studies showed that intravenous infusion of OXT significantly increases thresholds for visceral perception in IBS patients (Louvel et al., 1996).

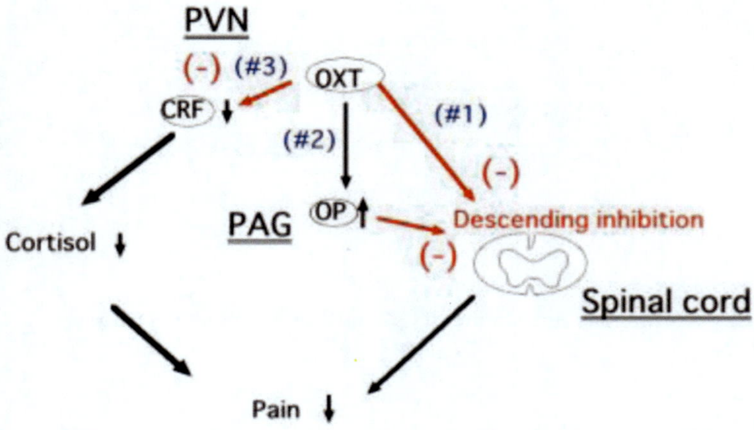

Figure 7.3. The possible mechanisms of anti-nociceptive effects of hypothalamic OXT. A direct descending projection of OXTergic neurons from the PVN to spinal cord and modulation of spinal dorsal horn neurons (#1; spinal pathway). A descending projection of OXTergic neurons from the PVN to PAG to enhance opioid (OP) release (#2; ponto-medullary pathway). OXT-induced inhibition on CRF release and reduction of systemic cortisol (#3; CRF-HPA axis pathway).

5. Cardiovascular Effects

OXT has both central and peripheral actions on cardiovascular function (Petersson, 2002). Functional OXT receptors have been discovered in the rat and human heart, as well as in vascular beds (Jankowski et al., 2000). The cardiovascular activities of OXT may include: lowering blood pressure, parasympathetic neuromodulation, vasodilatation, anti-inflammatory, anti-oxidative, and metabolic effects. These effects are mediated, at least in part, by stimulating cardio-protective mediators, such as nitric oxide (NO) and atrial natriuretic peptide (ANP). OXT has the capacity to generate cardiac myocytes from various types of stem cells (Gutkowska et al., 2012).

OXT increases glucose uptake in cultured cardiac myocytes. In rats with experimentally-induced myocardial infarction, continuous *in vivo* OXT delivery improves the cardiac healing process, reduces inflammation and stimulates angiogenesis (Ondrejcakova et al., 2009; Wsol et al., 2009). Therefore, in pathological conditions, OXT exerts anti-inflammatory and cardio-protective properties, and improves vascular and metabolic functions (Gutkowska et al., 2012).

Daily administration of OXT for 5–14 days reduced blood pressure (Petersson et al., 1999; Holst et al., 2002). Massage-like stroking also caused blood pressure reductions via enhancing endogenous OXT activity (Petersson et al., 1999; Holst et al., 2002). Enhanced OXT activity leads to inhibition of central and peripheral adrenergic and HPA axis activity, while promoting parasympathetic cardiac control (Gutkowska et al., 2000; Mukaddam-Daher et al., 2001).

6. OXT Release in Response to Somato-sensory Stimulation

In primates, social grooming and allogrooming (the grooming of others) play an important role in social bonding. There are many pieces of evidence that OXT is associated with physical touch. In rats, high doses of OXT give rise to a sedative-like effect, including lowered blood pressure and reduced locomotion (Uvnas-Moberg, 1998a). The physical stimulation of suckling itself produces anti-stress effects that include a lowered blood pressure and a decreased sympathetic tone (Uvnas-Moberg, 1996, 1998a), similarly to those produced by social grooming.

Agren et al. (1995) reported that massage-like stroking of the abdomen raised plasma OXT levels in rats. This was associated with enhanced tolerance of pain (Agren et al., 1995). A recent study showed that acupuncture stimulates OXT expression at the PVN in rats (Yoshimoto et al., 2012a). In women, frequency of physical contact (hugs) with partners was correlated with elevated OXT levels and lowered blood pressure (Light et al., 2005). Fifteen minutes of moderate pressure massage increased plasma OXT levels after being trusted and increased reciprocity, compared to untouched controls (Morhenna et al., 2008).

Summary

OXT plays a critical role in the cause and effect of positive social interaction, resulting in a general feeling of mental and psychological well-being. OXT release is augmented by emotional and physiological support. The beneficial effects of manual therapies (acupuncture and massage), music therapy, and meditation are mediated via OXT release in the brain. The better understanding of the pathophysiological role of OXT may contribute to the development of integrative medicine.

Chapter 8

SOCIAL INTERACTIONS AND HEALTH

Social support is reliably related to beneficial effects on aspects of the cardiovascular, endocrine, and immune systems. Social support may have stress-buffering effects and emotional support appears to be an important dimension of social support (Uchino et al., 1996).

Our survival depends on the ability to build mutually beneficial relationships with others. It is important for us to feel connected, to be trusted and loved. Feeling connected to others increases psychological and physical well-being and decreases the risk of depression and physical ailments. A sense of connectedness also increases empathetic responding as well as acts of trust and cooperation. Social interactions have a profound effect on health. People with a higher quality of social relationships show a lower risk of death (Seeman, 1996), while social isolation has been shown as a major risk factor for mortality (House et al., 1988). Unfortunately, despite the clear benefits of social connectedness, our society is becoming increasingly isolated and distrustful.

1. ENVIRONMENT AND LONGEVITY

There are places around the world where people live longer and are active past the age of 100 years. The people living in these areas share common behavioral characteristics. These places (Sardinia in Italy, Okinawa in Japan, Loma Linda in California, and Nicoya Peninsula in Costa Rica) have been named the "Blue Zones". Recently it was reported that people on Ikaria Island, Greece, have also one of the highest life expectancies in the world, and this island joined the list of "Blue Zones" (Figure 8.1). On Ikaria Island, the majority of the oldest participants reported daily physical activities, healthy eating habits, and frequent socializing (Panagiotakos et al., 2011). The interaction of environmental and behavioral patterns may be key factors for longevity.

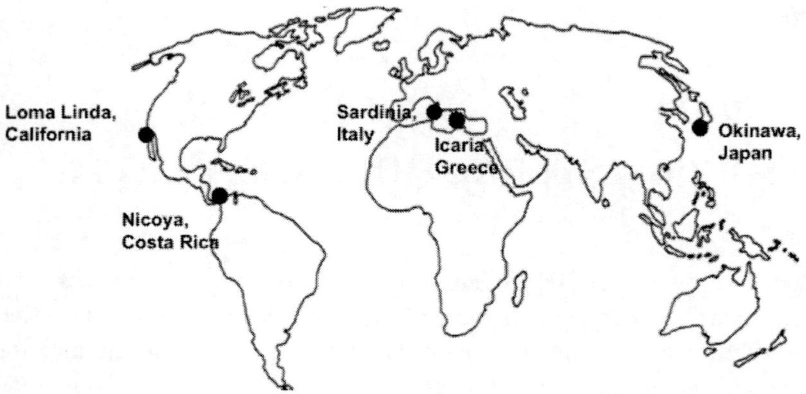

Figure 8.1. Blue zones in the world

2. Social Activity and Health

These are known as the Triple Jewels in Buddhism (Buddha, Dharma and Sangha). Dharma means "*teachings of the Buddha*" and Sangha means "*harmonious community*". Buddha, Dharma and Sangha together possess qualities that are precious like jewels and can lead one to enlightenment (The Teaching of Buddha).

Prospective studies consistently show an increased risk of death among people with low quantity and quality of social relationships. Experimental and quasi-experimental studies of humans and animals also suggest that social isolation is a major risk factor for mortality from widely varying causes (House et al., 1982).

In a study of middle-aged men, social influences, outside-home activities, and social activities at the baseline examination were found to be significantly associated with mortality. The association between these variables and mortality was significant even when age, risk factors for coronary heart disease, and health status measured at the baseline examination were taken into consideration. Thus, social activities may have a modifying effect on life stresses and risk factors associated with mortality (Welin et al., 1985).

People who lacked social and community ties were more likely to die than those with extensive contacts. The most important protective factors among men were married status and frequent contacts with close friends and relatives. These factors acted independently of self-reported health and habits such as smoking and alcohol consumption (Berkman et al., 1979).

Studies have shown that people with a higher quality of social relationships are shown to be at a lower risk of death (Seeman, 1996), while social isolation has been shown as a major risk factor for mortality (House et al., 1988). Access to a supportive family and social network has been shown to promote human health (Uvnas-Moberg, 1997b; Carter, 1998). Recent animal studies provide vital information that positive social interactions play an important role in the regulation of GI functions associated with stress in rats (Babygirija et al., 2010; Babygirija et al., 2012a).

3. Compassion and Empathy

As described in Chapter III, Buddhist traditions have emphasized the importance of cultivating connection and love toward others through techniques such as loving-kindness meditation (LKM). This practice, in which one directs compassion and wishes for well-being toward real or imaginary others, is designed to create changes in emotion, motivation, and behavior in order to promote positive feelings and kindness toward the others (Salzberg, 1995).

LKM is a mind-training practice to cultivate positive emotions, such as friendliness, warmth, caring, and compassion (Salzberg, 1995). Practitioners of LKM are taught to generate feelings of warmth and compassion toward a loved one, a neutral acquaintance, a stranger, and a hostile person (Salzberg, 1995). Through this practice of providing empathy and compassion toward others, feelings of anger, resentment, and anxiety can be released.

Randomized clinical research has demonstrated that the practice of LKM decreased chronic low back pain, psychological distress, anger (Carson et al., 2005). LKM also increased social connectedness (Hutcherson et al., 2008). There is also evidence that through the cultivation of positive emotions with LKM practice, individuals experience decreased illness symptoms as well as an increase in a broader range of personal resources such as social support, purpose in life, and increased mindfulness (Fredrickson et al., 2008), which predicted greater life satisfaction and reduced symptoms of depression.

In LKM, the practitioner focuses on the intention that another person experiences safety, health, peace, happiness, and freedom from suffering and its causes. Mortality was significantly reduced for individuals who reported providing instrumental support to friends, relatives, and neighbors, and individuals who reported providing emotional support to their spouse (Brown et al., 2003). Thus, it is highly conceivable that giving compassion and empathy to others may be beneficial for the givers.

4. Volunteering

It is likely that those individuals who are best adapted to their environment will be most likely to survive and reproduce and that their genetic characteristics will become more prevalent in the species in succeeding generations. This would be interpreted to mean that individuals who are the most selfish will be the most likely to survive (Dovidio et al., 2006).

Against this argument, however, studies of humans and other social animals showed widespread evidence of the beneficial effects of prosocial and altruistic behavior. Numerous studies reveal protective effects of volunteering on mental and physical health. Both consistency of volunteering over time and diversity of participation are significantly related to well-being and self-reported health. Participation in clubs and volunteer activities had a significant protective effect on mortality. Piliavin (2007) insisted that "one does well by doing good" (Piliavin et al., 2007).

What is the bio-psychological evidence of this concept? Based on the recent findings (Babygirija et al., 2012a), it is proposed that giving affection and empathy to others is a key factor in upregulating hypothalamic OXT expression. As OXT is linked to health promoting cardiovascular, analgesic, and anti-stress effects, upregulated OXT expression would help to maintain our mental and physical health.

5. OXT and Social Interaction

Social isolation is known to be a potent stressor. In juvenile prairie voles, social isolation during post weaning increases CRF and cortisol levels (Ruscio et al., 2007). Social isolation followed by an acute stressor is associated with increased CRF, ACTH and cortisol in adult male prairie voles (Grippo et al., 2007). On the other hand, paired housing in adult male and female mice before and after stroke was shown to decrease ischemic damage and thereby improving the behavioral outcome (Craft et al., 2005).

Besides its well-known physiological functions, OXT plays an important role in regulating social behavior and positive social interactions (Neumann, 2008). Centrally administered OXT induces partner preference and accelerates the formation of social contact in both male and female prairie voles (Cho et al., 1999).

HPA axis plays a major role in initiating stress-responses, and hypothalamic OXT reduces the activity of HPA axis. There was a recurrent association between high levels of activity in the HPA axis and the subsequent expression of social behaviors and attachments. Positive social behavior reduces HPA axis activity, while negative social interactions can have the opposite effect. Social interactions and attachment involve endocrine systems capable of attenuating HPA axis activity and modulating the autonomic nervous system (Carter, 1998).

Well-being is a state of absence of mental and physical disease and also of positive emotions and contentment. As OXT release is augmented by touch and physiological support, so the hormone is involved in both the cause and benefit of social interactions. Conceivably, frequent socializing may reduce depression rate via upregulated OXT expression.

5.1. Empathy and OXT

During the process of mammalian evolution, animals developed sympathetic neural and behavioral systems. Altruism can be considered morally virtuous and has been associated with empathy. The experience of empathy has been shown to motivate prosocial behaviors, such as volunteering and donations to charities (Dovidio et al., 2006). Psychologists have distinguished between empathy and distress as motivators to help others. These affective states lead to divergent motivations to help others. Those who experience distress are motivated to reduce their own aversive state, while those who experience empathy are focused on relieving the aversive state of another (Barraza et al., 2009). By assessing the effectiveness of psychotherapy and its curative factors, Bachar (1998) demonstrated that empathy is one of the most important techniques that lead to therapeutic success (Bachar, 1998).

A positive social interaction is bidirectional, involving both giving and receiving empathy/care. It is reasonable that receiving empathy from others may promote OXT expression, resulting in coping with chronic stress (Babygirija et al., 2010; Babygirija et al., 2012a). In addition, a recent animal study suggests that giving affiliation toward others upregulates hypothalamic OXT expression, which in turn attenuates stress responses (Babygirija et al., 2012a). It should be noted that providing social support is more beneficial than receiving it to reduce mortality in humans (Brown et al., 2003).

Behavioral correlations, such as an increase in generosity, have been reported following positive social interaction in humans (Barraza et al., 2009). Empathy toward strangers increased plasma OXT levels. Higher levels of empathy were also associated with more generous monetary offers toward strangers (Barraza et al., 2009). Barraza and Zak (2009) provided the evidence that OXT is a physiologic signature for empathy. Empathy significantly increased plasma OXT levels. Higher levels of empathy were associated with more generous monetary offers toward strangers (Barraza et al., 2009).

5.2. Upregulation of Endogenous OXT Expression

Even if intranasal spray of OXT (Kosfeld et al., 2005) is shown, in the near future, to have a beneficial effect on our daily life stress, the therapeutic indication of OXT spray is questionable. When OXT is administered daily, desensitization of OXT receptors and/or downregulation of endogenous OXT synthesis might be developed. It is highly recommended to upregulate the endogenous OXT system in our body (hypothalamus), rather than depending on exogenous OXT.

It should be emphasized that access to a supportive family and social network, which upregulates hypothalamic OXT expression (Uvnas-Moberg, 1997b; Carter, 1998), is an important factor to overcome daily life stress. During the process of maintaining the positive social interaction, both of giving and receiving empathic affiliation, OXT system is upregulated in our brain. Especially, thinking about helpless people and giving sympathy to them may upregulate hypothalamic OXT expression, which promotes mental and physical health of the givers. It remains to be studied whether the activation of PFC and/or ACC are involved in mediating hypothalamic OXT expression in response to social interaction, in the same way as mind-body therapies.

5.3. Social Interactions and Religion - Interpretation of Religious Thoughts

> "Blessed are the merciful, for they will be shown mercy"
> (New Testament).

Human health is prompted by access to a supportive family and social network (Uvnas-Moberg, 1997b; Carter, 1998). Volunteering activity demonstrates protective effects of on mental and physical health (Piliavin et al., 2007).

Enhanced OXT activity is a logical candidate to be one of the primary physiological mediators of the health benefits of emotional and physical support, particularly those linked to warm touch. The mechanism of beneficial effects of social contact may involve hypothalamic OXT expression.

> "You have heard that you should love your neighbor. But I say to you. Love your enemies and pray for them which persecute you" (New Testament).

Why should we love our enemies and pray for them? Our interpretation of Jesus' words is that giving empathy to others upregulates hypothalamic OXT expression, promoting and maintaining our well-being. Thus, empathy and goodwill toward anybody, your enemy as well as your neighbor, allows one to maintain mental and physical health through upregulated OXT expression.

Once a king went to see an old hermit and asked, *"What is the most important Buddhist teaching?"* The hermit answered, *"Do no evil, do only good. Purify your heart."* The king had expected to hear a very long explanation. He protested, "*But even a five-year old child can understand that*" "*Yes*," replied the wise sage, "*But even an 80-year-old man cannot do it.*" (The Teachings of Buddha).

Why should we "do good"? The understanding of Buddhist teaching is that committing acts of kindness toward others promotes upregulation of hypothalamic OXT expression, which spontaneously maintains our health.

Muslims appreciate the mercy and love of Allah.

> "When they have purified themselves, then come to them from where Allah has ordained for you. Indeed, Allah loves those who are constantly repentant and loves those who purify themselves" (Quran).

In order to receive the mercy and love of Allah, we need to purify ourselves. The interpretation of "to purify ourselves" is to maintain a positive social interaction including affection, empathy, and compassion to others.

> "If you want others to be happy, practice compassion. If you want to be happy, practice compassion." (Dalai Lama).

Buddhist traditions have emphasized the importance of cultivating connection and love toward others through techniques such as loving-kindness meditation (LKM) (Salzberg, 1995). The practice of LKM decreased chronic low back pain, psychological distress, and anger (Carson et al., 2005). Thus, it is important to reconsider Buddhist traditions of cultivating connection and compassion toward others in order to maintain our well-being.

SUMMARY

OXT has been implicated in a number of social behaviors, including affection and social attachment. A positive social interaction (both of receiving and giving care/empathy), which upregulates endogenous (internal) OXT expression, is an important factor to overcome our daily life stress. Especially, thinking about helpless people and giving compassion/empathy to them may upregulate OXT expression, which promotes mental and physical health.

Religious thoughts have emphasized the importance of cultivating connection and love toward others. As social interaction is a key factor to overcome daily life stress, the future medicine should emphasize every patient to improve their social ties.

Chapter 9

APPLICATION OF INTEGRATIVE MEDICINE FOR VARIOUS DISEASES

Integrative medicine can help resolve problems along with conventional Western medicine (CWM) and improve the circumstances of complementary and alternative medicine (CAM), thereby integrating the efficacy of CWM and CAM.

It is likely that the beneficial effects of CAM are mainly due to (1) the reduction of stress responses (anti-stress effects) and (2) the reduction of pain pathway (anti-nociceptive effects). Meditation and its related procedures may promote these effects by stimulating activity in the brain (especially, PFC and ACC) and throughout its network, while manual therapies may promote these effects via stimulating somatosensory activation. Both pathways finally activate the release of opioids and oxytocin (OXT) from the periaqueductal gray (PAG) and paraventricular nucleus (PVN), respectively. Released opioids and OXT mediate anti-nociceptive effects and anti-stress effects.

Thus, meditation and its related procedures may utilize PFC and ACC activation to stimulate PAG and OXT (top-down pathway), while manual therapies may utilize somatosensory activation to stimulate PAG and OXT (bottom-up pathway). In concert with both pathways, CAM is effective in various diseases associated with stress and pain. In addition, CAM can regulate the autonomic nervous system through both pathways (Figure 9.1). The enhancement of parasympathetic activity may be beneficial for GI diseases and cardiovascular diseases.

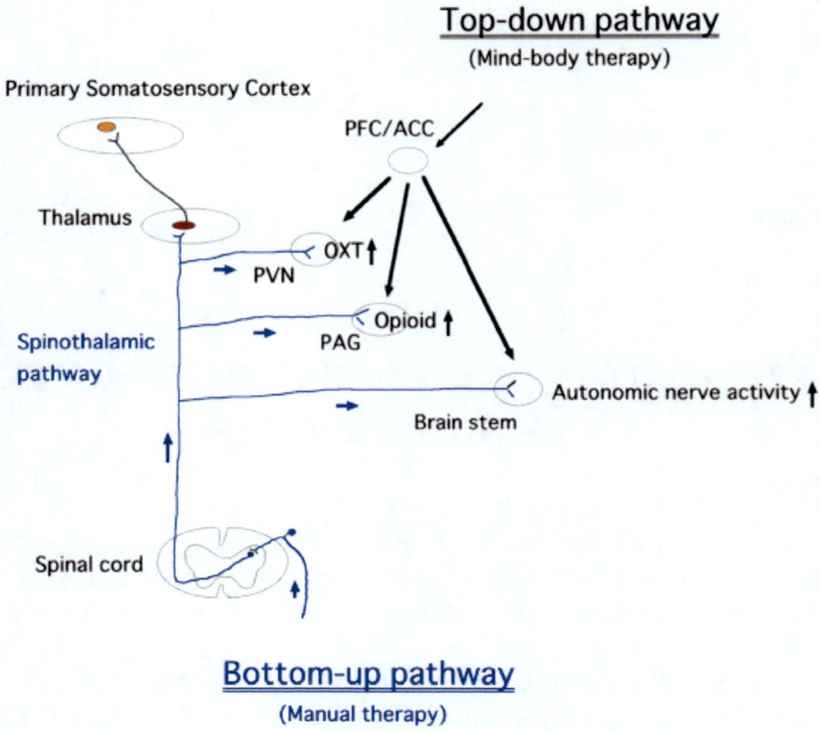

Figure 9.1. Mind-body therapies stimulate opioid release from the PAG and OXT release from the PVN, via the activation of PFC and ACC. These procedures also stimulate brain stem to regulate autonomic nervous function (top-down pathway; black lines). In contrast, manual therapies stimulate the PAG, PVN, and brain stem, via the activation of somatosensory pathways (bottom-up pathway; blue lines). Altered autonomic nervous function can improve the imbalance between the parasympathetic nerves and sympathetic nerves.

1. Anxiety Disorders

As described in Chapter III, stress affects the mind, body, and behavior. Stress stimulates corticotropin releasing factor (CRF) at the PVN, which promotes the release of adrenocorticotropin hormone (ACTH) from the anterior pituitary. Released ACTH stimulates the cortisol release from the adrenal grand. This pathway is called as hypothalamic-pituitary-adrenal (HPA) axis (Figure 3.7).

Major depression is associated with perturbations in social attachments, dysregulation of the HPA axis, and elevated levels of anxiety. For anxiety disorders, patients are often given supportive medications such as selective serotonin reuptake inhibitors (SSRIs) and diazepam (a minor tranquilizer). However, the shift amongst some health consumers toward alternate healing methods for depression, such as mind-body medicine, reflects both a belief in their therapeutic promise and growing interest in self-applied health interventions (Little et al., 2009). Data from a national health survey found a high use of CAM treatments for treating emotional distress with self-reported severe depression and anxiety (Kessler et al., 2001). Fifty four % of women with diagnosed depression used CAM in a 12-month period as a principal treatment for mood and emotional distress (Wu et al., 2007).

1.1. Pharmacological Treatment

Many depressed individuals tend to reject antidepressant medications for medical and personal reasons, such as long-term safety concerns, health contraindications, dissatisfaction with relapse rates (Segal et al., 2003), and suboptimal symptom relief (Williams et al., 2000; Hirschfeld et al., 2002). A meta-analysis of empirically supported psychotherapies showed improvement for 50% of depressed patients (Elkin et al., 1989), with typically more residual symptoms than for antidepressants (Westen et al., 2001).

This reality led to the development of alternative treatment options for depression, from combined therapy–medication group protocols to application of meditative techniques to psychotherapy. In our future medicine, anxiolytic agents such as SSRIs or diazepam may not be the first choice to treat anxiety disorders associated with stress, as far as CAM procedures (meditation, Yoga, Tai-chi, exercise, and acupuncture, etc.) are able to reduce symptoms.

1.2. Meditation

Currently, many patients are turning to meditation as an alternative approach to reduce stress and anxiety. Meditation offers a therapeutic and often spiritual approach that avoids side effects of medications and the stigma of psychiatric treatments.

Meditation is a whole package of mind–body exercise with possibility of change in life style or attitude, which includes both specific and non-specific effects. The potential regulatory functions of meditation practices on attention and emotion processes have a long-term impact on the brain and behavior.

Prefrontal cortex (PFC) is involved in working memory, decision making, planning and behavioral flexibility, as well as in social interactions and emotional processing. PFC intelligently regulates these functions through extensive connections with other brain regions. PFC is very sensitive to the detrimental effects of stress exposure. Even quite mild acute uncontrollable stress can cause a rapid and dramatic loss of prefrontal cognitive abilities, and more prolonged stress exposure causes architectural changes in prefrontal dendrites (Cerqueira et al., 2008; Arnsten, 2009). Therefore, the malfunctioning of PFC induced by prolonged stress is highly relevant to mental and physical health (Arnsten, 2009).

It has been shown that PFC is activated by various types of meditation, such as mindfulness meditation (Farb et al., 2007; Farb et al., 2012), Tibetan Buddhist meditation (Baron Short et al., 2007), and Zen meditation (Yu et al., 2011) (See Chapter III). Activation of the anterior PFC and serotonin (5-HT) system may be responsible for the improvement of negative mood observed during focused attention (FA) on abdominal breathing (Yu et al., 2011). Stress reduction is associated with slow, deep, regular, and diaphragmatic-abdominal breathing during meditation (Chapell, 1994).

Loving-kindness meditation (LKM) is a mind-training practice used to cultivate positive emotions, such as friendliness and compassion (Salzberg, 1995) (See Chapter III). The practice of LKM has significant beneficial effects, such as reduced psychological distress, reduced anger, and increased social connectedness (Carson et al., 2005; Hutcherson et al., 2008). There is also evidence that through the cultivation of positive emotions with LKM practice, individuals experience decreased illness symptoms as well as an increase in a broader range of personal resources such as social support, purpose in life, and increased mindfulness (Fredrickson et al., 2008), which predicted greater life satisfaction and reduced symptoms of depression.

1.3. Yoga

Yoga has been shown to have psychological effects: decreasing anxiety (Shelov et al., 2009) and increasing feelings of emotional, social, and spiritual well-being (Williams et al., 2005). Yoga also reduced sleep disturbances following 6 months of practice in a geriatric population (Manjunath et al., 2005). Self reported state anxiety and trait anxiety were significantly decreased in Yoga group compared to the control group (Rao et al., 2009). Women with metastatic breast cancer showed less pain and fatigue and increased relaxation after one year of weekly Yoga (Carson et al., 2007). In breast cancer patients, weekly Yoga sessions similarly led to improved quality of life and reduced anxiety (Speed-Andrews et al., 2010; Ulger et al., 2010).

The psychological effects of Yoga are mediated via down-regulation of HPA axis and the sympathetic nervous system. Studies showed that Yoga decreases levels of salivary cortisol (West et al., 2004; Michalsen et al., 2005) and urine catecholamine levels (Selvamurthy et al., 1998), resulting in reduced heart rate and systolic and diastolic blood pressure (Selvamurthy et al., 1998; Damodaran et al., 2002; Gokal et al., 2007).

1.4. Tai-chi

Tai-chi has been shown to reduce cortisol levels (Lee et al., 2004). Slater and Hunt (1997) reported a decrease in nightmares after Tai-chi exercise, as compared to a stretching exercise control group (Slater et al., 1997). In older adults, a 6-month Tai-chi program improved moderate sleep complaints. Thus, Tai-chi appears to be effective as a non-pharmacological approach to sleep enhancement for sleep-disturbed elderly individuals (Li et al., 2004). Incorporating Qi-gong and Tai-Chi can support the potential efficacy for survivors of torture and refugee trauma (Grodin et al., 2008).

Tai-chi has been shown to acutely decrease sympathetic nerve activity (Motivala et al., 2006). After Tai-chi practice, the parasympathetic activity increased, while sympathetic activity decreased. Heart rate, systolic blood pressure and diastolic blood pressure also decreased sequentially after Tai-chi. These suggest that Tai-chi enhances the vagal modulation and tilt the sympatho-vagal balance (Lu et al., 2003).

1.5. Physical Exercise

The effect of physical exercise on depressive state has been well demonstrated in adolescent females. Twenty-four hour excretions of cortisol and epinephrine in urine were reduced by exercise regimen (Nabkasorn et al., 2006). Exercise also stimulates the secretion of endogenous opioids and produces a state of euphoria (Grossman et al., 1984; Harber et al., 1984; Janal et al., 1984; Sher, 1998; Boecker et al., 2008). Exercise also promotes the secretion of neurotransmitters like 5-HT and dopamine (Ransford, 1982). The exercising rats showed less anxious behavior in the novelty situation. The changes in the sympatho-adrenomedullary input may play an important role in these distinct cortisol responses to stress (Droste et al., 2007).

Receptors or nerve fibers are excited and shows rhythmic discharges by strong muscle contractions induced by protracted exercise. This somato-sensory stimulation induced by exercise may be carried to the central nervous system (CNS), resulting in the release of endogenous OXT (Andersson et al., 1995). OXT has been shown to have anti-stress effects via inhibiting HPA-axis (Bulbul et al., 2011).

1.6. Acupuncture

Acupuncture needles are filiform, sterile, single-use needles that are thinner than insulin needles. Insertion of acupuncture needles causes minimal or no pain and much less tissue injury than phlebotomy or parenteral injection. Most side effects are minor, such as faintness, needle site bleeding, nerve damage, pneumothorax, and abortion in pregnant woman. Many patients find acupuncture treatment relaxing. The current expense and inconvenience of frequent visits to acupuncturists are the most common barriers to acupuncture treatment.

Although increasing numbers of patients are seeking acupuncture treatment for depression in recent years, the effectiveness of acupuncture remains unclear. Wu et al. (2012) conducted a PubMed search for publications through 2011. Acupuncture reduced side effects of anti-depressant in major depressive disorder. Published data suggest that acupuncture is a potential effective mono-therapy for depression, and a safe, well-tolerated augmentation in anti-depressant partial responders and non-responders (Wu et al., 2012). In addition to measuring clinical response, several clinical studies have assessed changes in levels of neurotransmitters and other biological response modifiers in an attempt to elucidate the specific biological actions of acupuncture (Pilkington, 2010). In contrast, others found insufficient evidence to recommend the use of acupuncture for people with depression (Smith et al., 2010).

The inserted needles are twisted manually or stimulated by electricity (electro-acupuncture; EA). Thus, the procedure may stimulate the somatic afferent nerves of the skin and muscles. As described in Chapter IV, some impulses of somatosensory stimulation are relayed to the brain stem, PAG and hypothalamus, via collateral connections (Hendelman et al., 2010).

Acupuncture can regulate autonomic function to stimulate the nucleus tractus solitarius (NTS), dorsal motor nucleus of vagi (DMV), and rostral ventrolateral medulla (RVLM) of the brain stem (Imai et al., 2009; Takahashi, 2011; Taniguchi et al., 2012). Acupuncture also stimulates opioid release from the PAG (Li et al., 2009) and OXT release from the hypothalamus (Yoshimoto et al., 2012a), respectively. Released opioid and OXT may work to suppress stress responses and anxiety (See Chapter IV and VII). Thus, anti-stress effects of acupuncture may be explained by its stimulatory effects on the autonomic nerves and OXT/opioid system (Figure 4.3).

1.7. Placebo Effects on Depression

In depression, there are clinical evidences that different regions of the brain linked to 5-HT are involved in the placebo response for depression. The placebo group manifests a mean therapeutic effect of 30%, while the active group manifested 50% (Walsh et al., 2002; Sysko et al., 2007). Recent meta-analyses evaluation of the clinical efficacy of antidepressant medications in the treatment of major depressive disorders concluded that there was no significant difference in comparison to placebo in the patients with moderate depression, and only a relatively small difference for patients with very severe depression (Kirsch et al., 2008; Fournier et al., 2010).

Leuchter et al. (2002) conducted a clinical trial with patients suffering from major depression, who were given antidepressants or placebo for 9 weeks. While the pre-treatment group presented no difference of brain activity, the placebo-responsive group manifested a significant increase of a strong correlation with the brain activity and cerebral perfusion at the PFC. This alteration was observed early in the treatment and not seen in either the non-responsive group or the antidepressant responsive group (Leuchter et al., 2002).

Using PET, Mayberg et al. (2002) studied the effects of anti-depressant (fluoxetine) and placebo. Remission of symptoms was observed in approximately half of each group. The placebo response was associated with an increased glucose metabolism in the PFC, parietal cortex, ACC, and posterior cingulate cortex (PCC). Subjects who responded to fluoxetine showed a similar metabolic pattern, suggesting a possible involvement of 5-HT in the antidepressant effects of placebo induction (Mayberg et al., 2002).

Central OXT seems to be involved in mediating placebo effects. As mentioned in Chapter VI, social interaction stimulates OXT release and that OXT mediates trust, analgesic and anti-depressive effects. It is conceivable that a reliable patient-doctor relationship increases OXT expression in the patients' brain, resulting in analgesic and anti-depressive effects. Further studies are needed whether the hypothalamic OXT stimulation is initiated via the activation of the PFC in response to a reliable patient-doctor relationship.

Enck et al. suggested that OXT is the central mediator of the placebo response (Enck et al., 2009). It is likely that emotional impact (whatever non-specific or psychological) can alter the brain activity, especially OXT neurons, which leads to the beneficial effects.

1.8. Depression and OXT

Plasma OXT levels are reduced in patients who are suffering from major depression (Frasch et al., 1995). Cyranowski et al. (2008) compared patterns of peripheral OXT release exhibited by depressed and non-depressed women. As compared with non-depressed controls, depressed women displayed greater variability in pulsatile OXT release. OXT concentrations were associated with greater symptoms of depression, anxiety and interpersonal dysfunction. Depressed women were more likely than controls to display a dysregulated pattern of peripheral OXT release (Cyranowski et al., 2008).

In animal models of depression, OXT has been shown to act as a potent anti-depressant (Arletti et al., 1987). One of the actions of SSRIs is through increased OXT release (Uvnas-Moberg, 1996; Uvnas-Moberg et al., 1999). Administration of SSRIs increased plasma OXT levels in rats (Uvnas-Moberg et al., 1999). OXT may regulate 5-HT release and exert anxiolytic effects via direct activation of OXT receptor expressed in 5-HT neurons of the raphe nuclei (Yoshida et al., 2009).

The inhibitory effect of OXT on CRF expression is mediated by $GABA_A$ receptors at the PVN (Bulbul et al., 2011). The anxiolytic agent, diazepam, is a $GABA_A$ receptor agonist. Subcutaneous administration of low dose of OXT has an anxiolytic effect in rats (Uvnas-Moberg et al., 1994). It is likely that the anxiolytic affect of OXT is mediated via $GABA_A$ receptors at the PVN (Bulbul et al., 2011). As described in Chapter III and IV, Yoga, acupuncture, massage, and aromathearapy are shown to stimulate OXT system. These therapies may be benefial to inhibit CRF and HPA axis activity in response to stress.

2. POSTTRAUMATIC STRESS DISORDERS (PTSD)

In humans, post-traumatic stress disorders (PTSD) are marked by deficits in anxiety, stress regulation and in social functioning. Traumatic stress in the normal individual results in activation of the sympatho-adrenal system causing a rise in noradrenaline/adrenaline, and activation of the HPA system resulting in elevated levels of cortisol. Studies in animals and in humans with PTSD indicate that chronic traumatic stress can result in dissociation of the sympatho-adrenomedullary and the HPA systems, resulting in sustained elevations of ACTH-cortisol responsivity (Wang, 1997). Cognitive behavioral therapy and pharmacotherapy have been used to desensitize and reprocess cognitions into clear emotional and physical plots that reformulate the traumatic experience.

2.1. Yoga

PTSD is highly prevalent among US military veterans. Mindful practices are widely offered in VA specialized PTSD treatment programs. Yoga, defined to include physical postures and mindfulness and meditation, is being increasingly used as an adjunctive treatment for PTSD.

Libby et al., (2012) assessed the prevalence, nature, and context of the use of yoga, mindfulness, and meditation in Department of Veterans Affairs' PTSD treatment programs. There was a great variability in the context and nature of how they are delivered. Therefore, the outcomes were not yet conclusive (Libby et al., 2012). Future studies are needed to assess the efficacy of CAM treatments, both as an alternative and as an adjunct to conventional PTSD treatment, and develop methods to tailor these treatments to veterans with PTSD.

2.2. Acupuncture

A recent clinical trial demonstrated that acupuncture is effective for treating the patients with PTSD. People diagnosed with PTSD were randomized to either an empirically developed acupuncture treatment or a group cognitive-behavioral therapy. Compared with the cognitive-behavioral therapy, acupuncture provided significant effects on PTSD. Symptom reductions observed at the time that acupuncture treatments ended, were maintained at 3-month follow-up (Hollifield et al., 2007).

Various types of somatosensory stimulations (grooming, touch, hug, massage, etc.) are useful to treat PTSD because of its stimulatory effects on OXT system (Uvnas-Moberg et al., 1993; Uvnas-Moberg et al., 2005; Yoshimoto et al., 2012a) (See Chapter VII). In addition, it is conceivable that acupuncture, massage, and TENS, all of which upregulate endogenous OXT expression, are effective for PTSD.

2.3. PTSD and OXT

A recent study suggested that OXT is a likely candidate for treatment of patients with PTSD through a reduction of fear response and an increase of social functioning (Olff et al., 2010). It has been suggested that OXT has unique effects of decreasing background anxiety without affecting learning and memory of a specific traumatic event in rats (Missig et al., 2010). Increased OXT neurotransmission during traumatic events is likely to prevent the formation of aversive memories. When OXT was centrally administered prior to fear conditioning or extinction training, fear expression and facilitated fear extinction were decreased in rats. The effect of OXT on fear extinction was abolished by OXT receptor antagonists. Thus, Toth et al. proposed that OXT treatment before fear extinction training is a comparable time point for psychotherapy in PTSD patients (Toth et al., 2012).

In humans, 3,4-methylenedioxymethamphetamine (MDMA; ecstasy) robustly induces OXT release (Johansen et al., 2009). Thus, MDMA in combination with psychotherapy may be beneficial for treatment-resistant anxiety disorders (Johansen et al., 2009). Stress-associated diseases such PTSD may be treatable by OXT and/or MDMA, administered in a diluted and strictly controlled fashion.

3. Chronic Pain

Pain is one of the most common reasons for seeking medical care. The prevalence of chronic pain in the general population ranges from 10% to over 40%. Patients with chronic pain use health services up to five times more than patients without pain (Von Korff et al., 1991). The estimates for the total cost of chronic pain exceed $210 billion annually in US (Turk et al., 2011).

For chronic pain, pharmaco-therapeutic options include opioid derivatives, acetaminophen, anti-inflammatory medications. These medications target inflammation and relieve pain. In contrast, the trend toward use of CAM therapies is quite common in patients with chronic pain. The survey of patients with chronic pain disorders conducted in 12 primary care clinics in USA found that 52% reported using CAM therapies to assist with pain relief (Rosenberg et al., 2008). Forty four % of primary care patients with chronic pain receiving opioid therapy had used CAM treatments in the last 12 months (Fleming et al., 2007). Other studies examining the use of CAM therapies for various chronic pain states report rates ranging from 35% to 63% (Lee et al., 2011).

The integration of non-pharmacologic interventions such as meditation, therapeutic exercise, manual therapies (acupuncture, massage, and TENS) are recommended and may provide a low-cost and minimal-risk option for patients to manage their diseases.

3.1. Pharmacological Treatments

Oral drugs have been the mainstay of treatment for pain during past centuries, and the use of drugs to treat pain has expanded exponentially in recent years, with increases in expenditures of 188% between 1996 and 2005 (Martin et al., 2008).

3.1.1. Opioid

Retail sales for opioids, the most common class of drug prescribed in the USA, increased by 176% from 1997 to 2006. However, their use remains controversial both with respect to efficacy and adverse physical effects (Stein et al., 2010).

A meta analysis of 41 randomised controlled trials evaluating the effectiveness of opioids for the treatment of chronic pain demonstrated that opioids result in a small improvement in pain severity and functional improvement compared with placebo (Furlan et al., 2006). Notably, the placebo response rate for opioid trials is around 10%, and when active placebos that mimic the side effects of opioids are used, the response rate increases to an average of 21% (Turk, 2002). This suggests that setting of realistic expectations with patients is crucial.

Side effects associated with opioids are nausea, constipation, and somnolence. In addition, a few patients with long-term opioid treatment can develop opioid-induced hyperalgesia: when patients taking opioids become hypersensitive to nociceptive stimuli (Chu et al., 2008). Thus, opioids can be recommended as the second- or third-line treatment (Attal et al., 2010; Turk et al., 2011).

3.1.2. Non-Steroidal Anti-Inflammatory Drugs

The efficacy of non-steroidal anti-inflammatory drugs (NSAIDs) has been reported for patients with osteoarthritis, rheumatoid arthritis and back pain (Roelofs et al., 2008). The most prominent members of NSAIDs are aspirin, ibuprofen, and naproxen. NSAIDs-induced gastropathy is regarded as one of the most common adverse effects (Griffin et al., 2001). Careful scrutiny for the development of adverse reactions should be undertaken, particularly with long-term use of NSAIDs. Selective cyclo-oxygenase (COX)-2 inhibitors have fewer gastrointestinal (GI) side effects than traditional NSAIDs, but they are associated with increased cardiovascular risk (Roelofs et al., 2008).

Although paracetamol (acetaminophen) is used to treat inflammatory pain, it is not generally classified as NSAIDs because it exhibits only weak anti-inflammatory activity. Paracetamol is a slightly weaker analgesic than NSAIDs, but is a reasonable alternative because of reduced gastrointestinal complications and low cost (Kroenke et al., 2009). The widespread use of paracetamol, combined with the small margin of safety between therapeutic and toxic dose, often result in an un-intentional overdose (Guggenheimer et al., 2011). On the basis of growing rates of un-intentional overdose and hepatic failure associated with paracetamol, the FDA revised the drug's warning label in April, 2010 (Turk et al., 2011).

3.2. Dietary Modifications

Anti-inflammatory diets can favorably influence the biochemical process of inflammation present in pain syndromes. Omega-3 fatty acids and omega-6 fatty acids are a family of poly-unsaturated fatty acids. Omega-6 fatty acids are converted into the pro-inflammatory agents, such as arachidonic acid (AA) and prostaglandins (PG), which cause the sensation of pain and expedites healing and immune response in traumatized and infected tissues (Kelley, 2001). In addition, omega-3 fatty acids compete with omega-6 fatty acids for the same enzymes (5-desaturase and elongase). Therefore, increased inflammation precursors can be achieved by increased ingestion of omega-6 fatty acids and/or increasing the ratio of omega-6/omega-3 fatty acids in the diet (Rennie et al., 2003) (Figure 9.2).

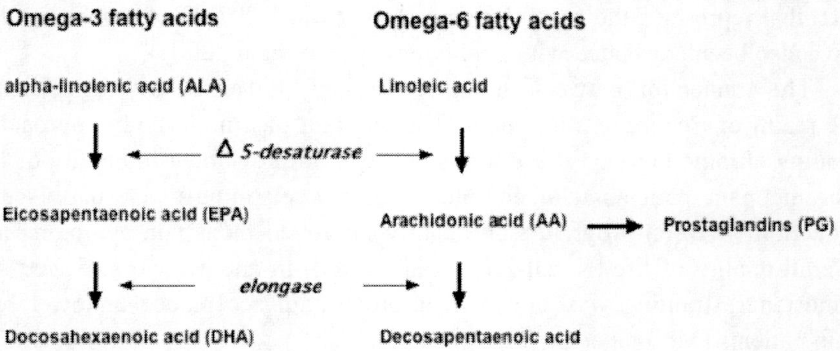

Figure 9.2. Omega-3 fatty acids compete with omega-6 fatty acids for the same enzymes (5-desaturase and elongase). Thus, increased inflammation precursors (AA and PG) can be achieved by increased ingestion of omega-6 fatty acids.

The ingestion of olive oil, a mono-unsaturated fatty acid, does not contribute to the omega-6 pool. Therefore, it can also reduce the omega-6/omega-3 ratio. Diets with less meat contribute less to the AA pool, which can diminish pro-inflammatory compounds. Fruits and vegetables contain phyto-chemicals which can act as anti-oxidants, reducing oxidative stress seen in pain conditions such as osteoarthritis.

Three major omega-3 fatty acids are available in foods: alpha-linolenic acid (ALA) eicosapentaenoic acid (EPA), and docosahexaenoic acid (DHA). EPA and DHA are found in cold-water fish such as salmon, mackerel, halibut, sardines, and herring. ALA is found in flaxseeds, flaxseed oil, canola (rapeseed) oil, soybeans, soybean oil, pumpkin seeds, pumpkin seed oil, purslane, perilla seed oil, walnuts, and walnut oil.

The Mediterranean diet is high in fruits, vegetables, fish, and mono-unsaturated fats (olive oil). The diet has a low intake of dairy products and red meat, and with the inclusion of omega-3, fish is an example of an anti-inflammatory diet (Teets et al., 2010).

3.3. Meditation

Centrally maintained pain has been correlated with cortical plasticity. The brain can undergo neurological changes with time in correlation with sensations of chronic pain (Flor et al., 1997; Knost et al., 1997). Several changes in the somatosensory cortex have been correlated in patients with chronic pain, including an enlarged area of activation in the part of the body map that represents the painful region (Kerr et al., 2007). These abnormalities have also been correlated with pain intensity (Flor et al., 2001).

The connection between the mind and body is particularly significant in the realm of treating chronic pain. The addition of a mind-body approach to treating chronic pain may lead to a significant improvement in quality of life. Chronic pain patients who completed an 8-week mindfulness-based stress reduction (MBSR) program significantly improved their pain symptoms and overall quality of life (Kabat-Zinn et al., 1985). In another work, 8 weeks of mindfulness training was shown to improve pain acceptance in lower back pain patients (Morone et al., 2008).

Garland et al. (2011) recently determined that 8 weeks of mindfulness training significantly improved pain symptoms in irritable bowel syndrome (IBS) patients, even after three months of training. Mindfulness meditation reduced pain symptoms by reducing anxiety and emotional reactions to IBS symptoms (Garland et al., 2011).

3.4. Yoga

After 3-4 months of Yoga sessions, back pain (Sherman et al., 2005; Williams et al., 2005), rheumatoid arthritis (Evans et al., 2010), and headache (John et al., 2007) were significantly reduced. Yoga participants after 12 weeks of weekly classes reported less pain killer use than the waiting list control group (Saper et al., 2009).

Yoga has also been effective for osteoarthritis of the hands and knees. After Yoga sessions for 8 weeks, the participants experienced less pain, and improved physical functions (Garfinkel et al., 1994; Kolasinski et al., 2005).

3.5. Acupuncture

Opioid-induced anti-nociception is mediated via a pathway from the PAG to various brain nuclei. Opioids are likely to exert direct effects on PAG projection neurons through both delta- and mu-opioid receptors (Wang et al., 2002a). It has been well demonstrated that the analgesic effects of acupuncture are mediated by an endogenous opioid pathway (Stux et al., 1995; Diehl, 1999). Acupuncture reduces visceral pain via a central opioid pathway (Iwa et al., 2005).

It is conceivable that EA impulses are relayed via collateral connections to the PAG, which contains the endogenous opioids. PAG sends inhibitory information to the spinal dorsal horn and blocks noxious signal inputs from the periphery (descending inhibition) (Figure 4.5, #1).

Others showed that electrical stimulation of peripheral nerves results in an inhibition to the pain pathways at the spinal cord level (Hanai, 2000), suggesting that acupuncture may inhibit the pain pathway at the spinal cord levels as well (Figure 4.5, #2).

In addition to opioids, hypothalamic OXT has anti-nociceptive effects (Stock et al., 1988; Uvnas-Moberg et al., 1993; Agren et al., 1995; Yang et al., 2007) (See Chapter VII). As mentioned earlier, somatosensory simulation is carried to the hypothalamus as well. Acupuncture can stimulate OXT expression at the PVN (Yoshimoto et al., 2012a), suggesting that anti-nociceptive effects of acupuncture is mediated by the combined effects of opioid and OXT (Figure 4.3).

3.6. Exercise

Among non-pharmacologic interventions, therapeutic exercise is the most studied and supported in the literature (Zhang et al., 2007; Fransen et al., 2009a; Fransen et al., 2009b). Exercise is an effective treatment for various chronic musculoskeletal pain disorders, including chronic low back pain (van Middelkoop et al., 2010), chronic whiplash associated disorders (Stewart et al., 2007; Teasell et al., 2010), osteoarthritis (Jansen et al., 2011).

As described in Chapter IV, somatosensory neurons are physiologically activated by strong muscle contractions induced by protracted exercise. Exercise produces rhythmic discharges in nerve fibers, and causes the release of endogenous opioids and OXT essential to the induction of functional changes in different organ systems. Thus, the exercise-induced analgesia is presumably due to the release of endogenous opioids from the PAG (Koltyn et al., 1998; Koltyn, 2000) and OXT from the hypothalamus (Breton et al., 2009; Rojas-Piloni et al., 2010), which activates supra-spinal nociceptive inhibitory mechanisms (Millan, 2002; Ray et al., 2007).

3.7. Placebo-Induced Analgesia

Placebo analgesia is partly mediated by the endogenous opioid system (Benedetti, 1996; Amanzio et al., 1999; Sauro et al., 2005). Among the modulating mechanisms of placebo analgesia, it is postulated that the expectation of lessening of pain stimulates production of endogenous opioids (Teixeira et al., 2010).

Placebo analgesia is typically preceded by greater activation of the PFC during anticipation of pain, an effect that predicts reductions in pain perception and activity in pain-related brain regions (Petrovic et al., 2011). Positive expectations concerning analgesia would stimulate the dorsolateral PFC, which would then simultaneously activate the medial PFC, the orbito-frontal PFC and the opioid system of the brain (PAG) (Fricchione et al., 2005). Both placebo and the opioid agonist activated specific areas of the brain (medial PFC, orbito-frontal PFC and PAG) (Petrovic et al., 2002). This suggests a direct relationship between the placebo-induced analgesia and the opioid-induced analgesia. Wager et al. (2004) observed a decrease in pain with the application of a placebo cream on the arms of patients subjected to electric shocks, coinciding with an increase in brain activity in the orbito-frontal PFC, dorsolateral-medial PFC, and PAG (Wager et al., 2004).

Similarly, spoken suggestion-induced placebo analgesia showed the decrease of neural activity in the thalamus, and ACC with a simultaneous increase in the lateral amygdale and PAG in patients with IBS (Price et al., 2007). Thus, it is likely that positive expectation activates endogenous opioids and pain-modulating brain networks, resulting in inhibition of pain pathways (Figure 3.10).

3.8. Herbs

Two common culinary herbs have been shown to contain anti-inflammatory properties, ginger and turmeric. Ginger has long been used in traditional medical practice to reduce inflammation. Ginger showed a significant effect on reducing symptoms of osteoarthritis of the knee, compared to placebo (Altman et al., 2001).

Turmeric has been used for centuries in Ayurvedic medicine (Hindu system of traditional medicine native to India) as a treatment for inflammatory disorders including arthritis. Some preliminary clinical research suggests that turmeric may improve symptoms of rheumatoid arthritis (Funk et al., 2006).

However, a recent review article demonstrated that the data are not suggestive enough to recommend such supplements. Ginger and turmeric are unlikely to have clear effect on chronic pain conditions (Teets et al., 2010).

4. Functional GI Diseases

Functional GI disorders include functional dyspepsia (FD) and IBS. FD, also known as upset stomach or indigestion, is characterized by chronic or recurrent pain in the upper abdomen, upper abdominal fullness, and feeling full earlier than expected when eating. FD can be accompanied by bloating, belching, nausea, or heartburn. IBS is diarrhea or constipation predominant, or they alternate. Onset of IBS is more likely to occur after an infection, or a stressful life event (Talley, 1994; Drossman, 2006).

Functional GI disorders are common in the general population, with a reported prevalence of 25-40%. Functional GI disorders are responsible for up to 40% of office consultations to gastroenterologists (Talley, 1994; Drossman, 2006). The burden of IBS is estimated to be $1.6-$10 billion in direct costs and $19.2 billion in indirect costs in US.

IBS and FD have no known organic cause. The motor dysfunction of GI tract and visceral hypersensitivity are considered especially important factors for IBS and FD etiology (Drossman, 2006; Van Oudenhove et al., 2010). Disorders of colonic motility may contribute to symptoms in constipation- or diarrhea- predominant IBS (Vassallo et al., 1992; Camilleri et al., 1999).

Pathogenesis of FD and IBS is highly associated with stress. GI symptoms may depend on the degree of strength, duration and accumulation of various types of mental and social stress. In addition, these disorders could also depend on how we adapt to the stressful events in our daily life. Epidemiological studies suggest considerable overlap between FD and IBS. About half of the FD patients fulfill the criteria for IBS (Corsetti et al., 2004). The possible explanation of the overlap is that the dysfunctions of upper and lower gut are due to the expression abnormality of OXT and CRF at the hypothalamus.

4.1. Pharmacological Treatment

The medical treatment for FD is intended to affect gastric acid, such as proton pump inhibitors (PPIs) and H_2 receptor antagonists. The treatment options for IBS, such as anti-diarrhea, laxatives and anti-spasmodics, are primarily used to target individual symptoms. Newer medications approved for IBS include 5-HT_3 receptor antagonists and chloride channel agonists (Gaman et al., 2009). Although pharmacological therapies may temporarily relieve symptoms, they are often costly and may result in negative side effects (Gaylord et al., 2011).

Animal studies demonstrated that stress-related changes in colonic motility are blocked by selective CRF_1 receptor antagonists (Tache et al., 2004a; Tache et al., 2004b). To treat IBS patients, selective CRF_1 receptor antagonists have been developed. The group at Mayo Clinic assessed whether modulation of central and CRF_1 receptors affected colonic transit and bowel function in female patients with diarrhea-predominant IBS (D-IBS). This randomized, double blind, placebo-controlled, 2-week study evaluated the effects of oral pexacerfont, a selective CRF_1 receptor antagonist, on GI and colonic transit. Pexacerfont failed to show any significant effects relative to placebo on colonic transit, gastric emptying, stool frequency, consistency, and ease of passage (Sweetser et al., 2009). Thus, the efficacy of CRF_1 receptor antagonist for IBS patients remains unclear.

4.2. Herbs

Digestive symptoms account for 10% of the use of herbal therapy. Daikenchuto (TU-100) is a traditional Japanese medicine (*Kampo medicine*) that has been used to treat adhesive bowel obstruction (Itoh et al., 2002). TU-100 is a mixture of extract powders from dried Japanese pepper, processed ginger, ginseng, and maltose powder. Intraduodenal and intrajejunal administration of TU-100 (0.5, 1.5, and 3.0 g) increased motility of the duodenum, proximal jejunum, and distal jejunum in conscious dogs in a dose-dependent manner (Jin et al., 2001). TU-100 has a clinically significant promotility effect in small bowel and ascending colon transit in healthy subjects. TU-100 appears to be safe and well tolerated and is a potential treatment for constipation-predominant IBS (C-IBS) and functional constipation (Manabe et al., 2010).

4.3. Acupuncture and TENS

Acupuncture has been used for treating FD and IBS (Chang et al., 2001; Wang, 2004; Takahashi, 2006; Tillisch, 2006). Dysfunction of GI motility, visceral hypersensitivity, and hyper responsiveness to stress are considered as important factors of functional GI disorders. The somatosensory stimulation induced by acupuncture is relayed to some brain nuclei, including the brain stem, PAG, and hypothalamus via collateral connections. When the nucleus tractus solitarius (NTS) at the brain stem is activated by acupuncture, GI motility is altered via the autonomic nerves (Iwa et al., 2006; Imai et al., 2009). Once the PAG and hypothalamus are stimulated by acupuncture, opioid and OXT are released, respectively (Tatewaki et al. 2004; Yoshimoto et al., 2012a). Released opioid and OXT mediate anti-nociceptive effect and anti-stress effect. Thus, acupuncture improves GI dysmotility and reduces visceral pain and stress responses (Figure IV-3). These may beneficial for patients with functional GI disorders (Takahashi, 2011).

In contrast to acupuncture, TENS is a non-invasive procedure (Sluka et al., 2003), in which electrodes are placed on the skin and stimulated by electricity. It has been shown that TENS applied to the acupuncture points (transcutaneous-EA) at the hands and lower legs improved GI symptoms in patients with FD (Liu et al., 2008). TENS is a possible alternative candidate therapy for the treatment of patients suffering from stress-related diseases. TENS is side effect-free and cost-effective. TENS can be effectively done at home, is portable, requires little time commitment, is easy to learn. TENS is a promising treatment for anxiety and/or GI disorders in any population of patients (Sallam et al., 2007) Further clinical and basic studies are needed whether no needle insertion procedure (TENS) has similar effects on the somoatosensory pathway, compared to the needle insertion procedure (acupuncture).

4.4. Hypnosis

Hypnotherapy has been demonstrated to have the capacity to normalize visceral sensitivity and modulate motility in GI tract (Prior et al., 1990b; Whorwell, 1990). Hypnosis had specific effects that substantially improved the symptoms of IBS patients. More than 50% average reduction in IBS severity, substantial reduction in anxiety and depression, improved quality of life, and good maintenance of symptom improvement were shown after the hypnosis treatment (Whorwell et al., 1984). Hypnosis is also effective in the long-term management of FD (Calvert et al., 2002).

OXT released in response to social stimuli may be part of a neuroendocrine substrate, which underlies the benefits of positive social experiences. Because of the special properties of OXT, including the fact that it can become conditioned to psychological state or imagery, OXT may mediate the benefits attributed to hypnosis therapy (Uvnas-Moberg et al., 2005; Bryant et al., 2012).

4.5. Meditation

A recent randomized controlled trial showed that mindfulness training reduces the severity of IBS in women. Women in the mindfulness group training showed greater reductions in IBS symptom severity at the 3-month follow-up relative to support group. Changes in quality of life, psychological distress, and visceral anxiety were also significantly improved in the mindfulness group training than the 3-month follow-up (Gaylord et al., 2011). Thus, mindfulness training has a substantial therapeutic effect on bowel symptom severity, improves health-related quality of life, and reduces distress.

4.6. Placebo Effects

A meta-analysis reviewing the placebo effect of several clinical trials for IBS in adults has found an average placebo response of 40% with a range of 16 to 71% (Patel et al., 2005). Studies on the placebo effect in adult patients with IBS showed that desires and expectations influenced placebo effects (Vase et al., 2005). The high placebo effect was the result of a high level of expectancy of the subjects and the parents. In addition, a strong family-doctor relationship was observed by a frequent contact between physician and subjects throughout the study (Saps et al., 2009). In IBS patients the patient–practitioner relationship is probably the most robust factor contributing to the placebo effect (Kaptchuk et al., 2008).

5. Cardiovascular Disease

Holistic integrative medicine is about treating all the risk factors for cardiovascular disease and getting to their underlying cause, whether it is sedentary lifestyle, hyperlipidemia, or maladaptive responses to stress. Although genetics accounts for approximately 20% of cardiovascular risk, 70% to 90% of chronic cardiovascular disease is related to an individual's lifestyle and environment.

The risk factors for cardiovascular disease are multifactorial. These risk factors range from hyperlipidemia, inflammation, diabetes mellitus, hypertension, and tobacco use to sedentary lifestyle and social connection. The psychological risks linked to cardiovascular disease include stress, anxiety, depression, and social isolation. Stress can adversely affect autonomic and vascular tone, immune function, coagulation, and the perception of pain. Anger increases the risk of myocardial infarctions by 230% (Mittleman et al., 1995).

Major depression, depressive symptoms, and anxiety significantly predicted cardiac events (Frasure-Smith et al., 1995b). Individuals with mental stress during daily life have twice the risk of myocardial ischemia. Depression is common after acute myocardial infarctions and is associated with an increased risk of mortality for at least 18 months. The patients with post-myocardial infarctions depression have higher mortality rates than non-depressed controls (Frasure-Smith et al., 1995a).

In a 5-year follow-up study, Blumenthal et al. (2005) demonstrated that stress management significantly reduced the risk of cardiovascular events compared with controls (Blumenthal et al., 2005). Psycho-educational programs demonstrated a 29% reduction in myocardial infarctions recurrence and a 34% reduction in overall cardiovascular mortality (Dusseldorp et al., 1999).

There are various non-pharmacological, mind-body therapies for dealing with and preventing cardiovascular diseases associated with stress. These therapies can be implemented in both the inpatient and outpatient care settings. Integrative medicine offers expertise in nutrition, exercise, and mind-body interventions that are pivotal to cardiovascular disease treatment and prevention. The approach to integrative cardiology includes nutrition counseling, cardiac rehabilitation (exercise), Yoga, meditation, acupuncture, and social support.

5.1. Dietary Modifications

The epidemiologic study evaluated the effect of nutrition on various diseases in rural China and US (Campbell et al., 1998). In the study of more than 10,000 individuals, the US fat intake was twice as high, fiber intake was 3 times lower, and animal protein intake was 90% higher. The heart disease death rate was 17-fold greater for men and 6-fold greater for women in US than China. However, Asian immigrants to the US reached the US level of heart diseases within 2 generations (Campbell et al., 1998).

Fats and carbohydrates are the major macronutrients affecting cardiovascular health. Fats are broken down into saturated, mono-unsaturated, and poly-unsaturated fatty acids. Saturated fatty acids contain no double bonds in their fatty acid chains and are typically solid at room temperature. They are the predominant fats in dairy products, red meat, and tropical oils, such as coconut oil. Saturated fats increase total cholesterol and low-density lipoprotein (LDL)- cholesterol. Overall, the intake of saturated fat is associated with an increase in the incidence of cardiovascular disease (Ascherio, 2002).

Replacement of saturated fat with mono-unsaturated or poly-unsaturated fats is associated with 10-fold greater decrease in risk (Hu et al., 1997). Mono-unsaturated fatty acids contain only 1 double bond in their fatty acid side chains. Foods rich in mono-unsaturated fat include olive oil, canola oil, many types of nuts, and avocados.

Mono-unsaturated fats have been associated with lower cardiovascular disease risk. This is best illustrated by the Mediterranean diet, which is high in mono-unsaturated fats, namely olive oil. The Mediterranean diet group experienced 49% fewer cardiovascular events, 62% fewer sudden deaths, and 51% fewer non-fatal myocardial infarctions, in comparison to the National cholesterol education program diet group (Singh et al., 2002).

5.2. Physical Exercise

Human studies demonstrated that chronic aerobic exercise regimens improve cardiovascular function in older people (Benjamin et al., 2004) and those with cardiovascular risk factors (Hambrecht et al., 1998), as well as healthy young subjects (Clarkson et al., 1999).

Mild oxidative stress can act as a stimulant of physiological anti-oxidant systems and as a trigger for various physiological adaptations (Gomez-Cabrera et al., 2008). Regular physical exercise delays the accumulation of free radical-mediated cell damage by improving the anti-oxidative protective mechanisms in the myocardium (Radak et al., 2005; Ji et al., 2006).

In patients after myocardial infarctions, percutaneous coronary intervention, or coronary artery bypass graft surgery, those who participate in a comprehensive exercise rehabilitation program have a 6-fold decrease in cardiac death compared with those patients who do not undergo cardiac rehabilitation (Taylor et al., 2004).

A provocative study looking at exercise vs angioplasty in patients with coronary artery disease determined by more than 75% stenosis on angiography showed that those who exercised daily had a lower cardiovascular event-free survival and equal angina symptom improvement (Hambrecht et al., 2004).

Despite these and many other findings showing the benefits of exercise, physicians reported spending an average of 8 minutes counseling their patients on lifestyle change at routine annual visits. Furthermore, fewer than 5% of physicians advise patients to engage in physical activity at least 6 days per week as recommended by national guidelines (Guarneri et al., 2009).

5.3. Yoga

After 2 month-Yoga training, the exercise-induced increase in heart rate and systolic blood pressure were significantly reduced (Madanmohan et al., 2004). Yoga group showed a significant decrease in heart rate and blood pressure and greater aerobic performance, than the control group (Telles et al., 2000). Following a daily Yoga practice (1 hr/day for 20 weeks), the participants had decreased blood pressure, blood glucose, cholesterol and triglycerides and improved subjective well-being and quality of life (Damodaran et al., 2002).

Following one year of Yoga training, serum cholesterol level was reduced by 23% in the Yoga group, while the standard treatment control group showed a 4% reduction. The serum LDL-cholesterol was also significantly decreased in Yoga group (26%), compared to control group (3%) (Yogendra et al., 2004).

After one year of weekly sessions, Yoga group had fewer anginal episodes, improved exercise capacity, decreased body weight and lower serum total cholesterol levels. Revascularization procedures (coronary angioplasty or bypass surgery) were less frequently required in Yoga group, and coronary angiography showed that more lesions regressed and fewer lesions progressed in the dietary change plus Yoga group (Manchanda et al., 2000).

5.4. Tai-chi

Tai-chi has been shown to acutely decrease sympathetic nervous system activity (Motivala et al., 2006). Tai-chi reduces cortisol levels (Lee et al., 2004). After Tai-chi practice, the parasympathetic activity increased, while sympathetic activity decreased. Heart rate, systolic blood pressure, and diastolic blood pressure also decreased sequentially after Tai-chi. These suggest that Tai-chi may enhance the vagal modulation and tilt the sympatho-vagal balance (Lu et al., 2003).

5.5. Acupuncture

There have been a number of clinical studies focused on the effectiveness of acupuncture to reduce blood pressure in essential hypertension. In 1975, Tam et al. found that acupuncture produced a significant reduction in systolic and diastolic blood pressure in 24 out of 28 patients with essential hypertension (Tam et al., 1975). Shortly after 30 minutes of acupuncture, both systolic and diastolic blood pressure were lowered by 10–20 mmHg in 50 patients with essential hypertension (Chiu et al., 1997), suggesting an immediate post-acupuncture effect.

After 6 week-treatment, acupuncture, but not sham acupuncture, significantly lowered mean 24-hr ambulatory blood pressures in 144 outpatients with un-complicated arterial hypertension (Flachskampf et al., 2007). Others also showed that acupuncture performed once weekly for 8 weeks, significantly reduced blood pressure. This beneficial effect appears to persist for a prolonged period of time (Zhou et al., 2012).

Acupuncture reduces blood pressure through modulation of the endocrine system, including decreases in plasma renin, aldosterone, and angiotensin II activity. Glutamate, acetylcholine, opioids, GABA, serotonin, nitric oxide (NO), and endocannabinoids in the brain all appear to participate in mediating anti-hypertensive response of acupuncture (Zhou et al., 2012).

5.6. Meditation

Transcendental meditation program was described as the principal mind-body technique, a comprehensive traditional system of natural medicine derived from ancient Vedic tradition in India (Schneider et al., 2005).

Transcendental meditation is a simple technique, which is practiced for 15-20 min twice daily. Transcendental meditation allows the mind to settle while alertness is maintained. The result is generally calm and clear thinking (Arthur et al., 2006).

Hypertension and cardiovascular morbidity/mortality were improved in patients who were taught transcendental meditation (Schneider et al., 2005). More recently, transcendental meditation has been shown to improve not only blood pressure but also the insulin resistance components of the metabolic syndrome as well as cardiac autonomic nervous system tone (Paul-Labrador et al., 2006)

5.7. Social Support

In a study of 887 post-myocardial infarctions patients, Frasure-Smith et al. (1995) found that 32% had mild to moderate depression. After 1 year, follow-up interviews were conducted and demonstrated that elevated depression scores were related to cardiac mortality. In contrast, higher levels of social support predict improvement in depression over the first post-myocardial infarctions year in those individuals with baseline depression and may protect patients from the negative prognostic consequences of depression (Frasure-Smith et al., 1995a). Thus, high levels of social support appear to decrease the magnitude of depression in post-myocardial infarctions patients (Guarneri et al., 2009).

6. Integrative Oncology

Cancer therapies of CWM include surgery, chemotherapy, and radiation. However, these may have side effects that seriously affect a patient's quality of life. Many people with cancer experience pain, anxiety, and mood disturbance. Conventional treatments do not always satisfactorily relieve these symptoms, and some patients may not be able to tolerate their side effects.

Cancer and its treatment typically evoke distress and emotional anguish. Patients experience fear of death, pain, disfigurement, disability, and many other distressing feelings. Depression is highly prevalent in cancer patients, where it is often under-diagnosed (Spiegel et al., 2003). These may fluctuate over time in response to various possible phases of the disease. Pharmacologic interventions such as anxiolytics and anti-depressants are effective in ameliorating these symptoms, although side effects or suboptimal relief are experienced by some patients.

The most frequently experienced side effects of chemotherapy are nausea and vomiting. Neuropathic pain usually does not respond to analgesics alone. Even with adjunct medications, many patients continue to experience this type of pain. Pain tends to become laced with anxiety and depression in patients faced with prolonged chronic pain, and these problems can affect caregivers as well as patients.

CAM such as acupuncture, mind-body techniques, and massage can relieve symptoms and improve physical and emotional well-being when used in conjunction with CWM. CAM can be used as low cost, convenient adjuncts to pharmacologic agents. Integrative medicine can be applied to alleviate the side effects of chemotherapy and radiation in the course of conventional cancer treatments (Dobos et al., 2012).

6.1. Meditation

CWM management of cancer-related symptoms (pain, nausea, fatigue, or sleep disturbance) typically involves pharmacological treatments, such as analgesics or sedatives. However, these medications may have unacceptable side effects or worsen some symptoms. In contrast, mind–body therapies have few or no negative side effects and may even improve symptoms in addition to the target symptom (Kwekkeboom et al., 2010).

Mind–body therapies provided for pain relief may also reduce anxiety and facilitate relaxation. Mind-body techniques can be particularly useful for patients who prefer active involvement and participation. Relaxation and imagery training can reduce pain and analgesic use, thus reducing analgesic side effects in some patients (Sloman et al., 1994; Syrjala et al., 1995).

A study of 115 cancer survivors utilizing Mindfulness-based cognitive therapy (MBCT) found improvements in depression, anxiety, distress, and mindfulness (Foley et al., 2010). MBCT is a purported refinement in mindfulness-based stress reduction (MBSR), which more specifically target the cognitive processes associated with relapse to depression. Improvements reported utilizing MBCT were moderate-to-large effect sizes and were maintained at a 3-month post-intervention follow-up (Foley et al., 2010).

Relaxation therapies minimize sympathetic nervous system response, which in turn decreases oxygen demand, slows heart rate, and lowers blood pressure. The mindfulness-based meditation therapies may have significant benefits for cancer survivors (Elkins et al., 2010).

6.2. Hypnosis

Clinical hypnosis can be defined as an altered state of consciousness, awareness, or perception (Stewart, 2005). Hypnosis is a highly relaxed state in which the patients' conscious and unconscious mind is open to therapeutic suggestion. Hypnotic relaxation is the most frequently cited form of non-pharmacological cognitive pain control. Hypnotherapy for the management of chronic pain has been demonstrated to provide relief for the symptoms of pain in cancer (Elkins et al., 2007).

Self-hypnosis can increase patients' feeling of self-efficacy and mastery of their internal and external environment (Jensen et al., 2006). In patients undergoing bone marrow transplantation, patients treated with hypnosis reported less oral pain (Syrjala et al., 1992). Breast-cancer patients utilizing self-hypnosis reported less pain and had increased duration of survival (Spiegel, 1983).

Self-hypnosis training for 15–20 min can reduce pain, fatigue, and discomfort in breast-cancer surgery patients. Patients undergoing excisional breast biopsy or lumpectomy received either a 15-min presurgery hypnosis session or empathic listening for the same duration of time. Those receiving the brief hypnosis session demonstrated significantly lower pain, discomfort, fatigue, and emotional distress postsurgery. In addition, those who received the hypnosis intervention needed less time in clinical care areas resulting in decreased institutional costs (Montgomery et al., 2010).

6.3. Yoga

A pilot study examined the effects of Yoga on a sample of 51 women with ovarian or breast cancer. All the women participated in 10 weekly Yoga classes, and upon completion of the study, the tabulated results showed subjective report of improvement in depression, negative affect, state anxiety, mental health, and quality of life (Danhauer et al., 2008). A randomized, controlled pilot study, evaluating Yoga in comparison with a waitlist control group, found improvements for mental health, depression, fatigue, positive affect, and spirituality on a sample of 44 breast cancer patients (Danhauer et al., 2009).

Duncan et al. (2008) examined the efficacy of a 6-week Yoga program in 24 cancer survivors, and found improvement in patient-reported quality of life, spiritual well-being, and mood (Duncan et al., 2008). After completion of a 12-week program, Yoga group showed improvement in quality of life and psychosocial functioning in breast cancer patients (Speed-Andrews et al., 2010).

The 8-week protocol involved gentle Yoga postures, breathing exercises, meditation, didactic presentations, and group interchange and led to decrease hot flashes in 37 breast-cancer survivors (Carson et al., 2009). Another pilot study of 13 women with metastatic breast cancer reported lower levels of pain and fatigue after participation in the Yoga of Awareness Program (Carson et al., 2007).

6.4. Tai-chi

In breast-cancer survivors, Tai-chi group showed a significant improvement in hand-grip strength, flexibility, and quality of life (Mustian et al., 2006). Effects of Tai-chi on anti-inflammatory and bone metabolism changes were tested in 16 breast cancer patients. Patients were randomized into either 12 weeks of 60-min Tai-chi sessions (3 times per week) or to the same schedule of standard support therapy. Compared to the standard support therapy, Tai-chi group had significantly increased levels of bone formation markers and IL-6 levels (Peppone et al., 2010).

6.5. Acupuncture

Acupuncture is well documented to relieve chronic cancer pain. A randomized, single-blinded, placebo-controlled trial tested auricular acupuncture for cancer patients who still experienced pain despite stable analgesic treatment. Ninety patients were randomized to one of three groups; needles placed at correct acupuncture points (treatment group), needles placed at non-acupuncture points, or application of pressure at non-acupuncture points (control groups). Pain intensity decreased by 36% at 2 months from baseline in the treatment group, a significant difference compared with the two control groups, where little pain reduction was seen (Alimi et al., 2000). As described in Chapter IV, the anti-nociceptive effect of acupuncture is mainly mediated via central opioid release (Stux et al., 1995; Diehl, 1999).

Acupoint of pericardium-6 (PC-6; hand) has been used for nausea and vomiting. Acupuncture at PC-6 decreases cisplatin-associated nausea and vomiting (Dundee et al., 1987). The recent review article concluded that acupuncture may alleviate chemotherapy-induced nausea and vomiting (Spencer et al., 2012). A clinical study also demonstrated that EA at PC-6 significantly inhibited the postoperative nausea and vomiting after the surgery (Dundee et al., 1989; Gan et al., 2004). Opioids have dual effects: an anti-emetic effect as well an emetic effect. It has been shown that central opioid plays a major role in mediating anti-emetic effect (Costello et al., 1977). Anti-emetic effect of acupuncture seems to be mediated via the central opioid pathway (Tatewaki et al., 2005) (See Capter IV).

Two single-arm pilot studies of acupuncture showed decreased mood disturbance associated with hormonal treatment in breast (Porzio et al., 2002) and prostate cancer patients (Hammar et al., 1999). A recent study suggests that anti-anxiety effect of acupuncture is mediated via the hypothalmic OXT release (Yoshimoto et al., 2012a).

Thus, anti-nociceptive effect, anti-emetic effects, and anti-anxiety effect of acupuncture are quite beneficial to treat the symptoms of cancer patients (Figure 4.3).

6.7. Massage

Randomized, controlled trials demonstrated that massage improves anxiety and other symptoms of distress. Massage therapy or reflexology (foot massage) may be beneficial for patients with chronic cancer pain and is increasingly available in hospital programs (Wilkie et al., 2000; Cassileth et al., 2004). This intervention is safe when given by properly trained massage therapists. Most patients feel better after massage therapy, and it may also result in substantial relief. Massage therapy also can enhance mood in patients with breast and lung cancer (Stephenson et al., 2000). However, the receipt of massage therapy is dependent on availability and economic factors.

6.8. Music Therapy

Music therapy is the clinical use of music interventions to accomplish individualized goals within a therapeutic relationship facilitated by a credentialed professional who has completed an approved music therapy program. Music therapy is a noninvasive and inexpensive intervention that appears to reduce mood disturbance in patients experiencing the stress of pending bone marrow transplantation (Cassileth et al., 2003). In a controlled study of music therapy for autologous stem-cell transplant recipients, there was lessened mood disturbance in response to the therapy, as compared to controls (Cassileth et al., 2003). In four studies of music therapy for the treatment of cancer-related chronic pain, music therapy demonstrates pre-to-post session reductions in pain (Cholburi et al., 2004). In contrast, two separate studies found no difference in reductions in pain when music listening was compared with controls (Kwekkeboom et al., 2010).

6.9. Herbs

Some patients use herbs for relief of anxiety, depression, and physical symptoms. These products are readily available as dietary supplements. Indeed, many botanicals contain biologically active substances that can effectively change mood or relieve pain.

Although the use of CAM by patients with cancer is high, patients frequently fail to disclose its use to their health professionals for reasons emanating from both sides of the dyadic patient-doctor relationship (Davis et al., 2012). As described in Chapter VI, there is a potential risk of herb-drug interactions. Patient-doctor communication about CAM is necessary to maintain patient safety and well-being.

It has been proposed that herbs and other botanical products should not be used during chemotherapy, or radiation, because they can interfere with prescription medications, alter coagulation, modulate the level and activity of drug-metabolizing enzymes, and produce herb-drug interactions (Deng et al., 2005).

SUMMARY

Integrative medicine can cover the current problems of CWM and improve the circumstances of CAM. The beneficial effects of CAM are mainly due to (1) reduction of stress responses (anti-stress effects) and (2) reduction of pain pathway (anti-nociceptive effects). Meditation and its related procedures may promote these effects via stimulating the PFC/ACC (top-down pathway), while manual therapies promotes these effects via stimulating somatosensory activation (bottom-up pathway).

Both pathways finally activate the release of opioids and OXT form the PAG and PVN, respectively. Released opioids and OXT mediate anti-nociceptive effects and anti-stress effects. In concert with both pathways, CAM is effective in various diseases associated with stress and pain. CAM also regulates autonomic nervous system through both pathways. The enhancement of parasympathetic activity is beneficial for GI diseases and cardiovascular diseases (Figure 9.1). Integrative medicine can be applied to alleviate the side effects of chemotherapy in the course of conventional cancer treatments.

REFERENCES

Aaron C., Lincoln T., 2003. The other drug war 2003: Drug companies deploy an army of 675 lobbyists to protect profits Washington (DC): Public Citizen Congress Watch. www.citizen.org/ documents/ Other_Drug_War2003.pdf

Agarwal S.K., Calaresu F.R., 1991. Monosynaptic connection from caudal to rostral ventrolateral medulla in the baroreceptor reflex pathway. *Brain Res* 555, 70-74.

Agren G., Lundeberg T., Uvnas-Moberg K., Sato A., 1995. The oxytocin antagonist 1-deamino-2-D-Tyr-(Oet)-4-Thr-8-Orn-oxytocin reverses the increase in the withdrawal response latency to thermal, but not mechanical nociceptive stimuli following oxytocin administration or massage-like stroking in rats. *Neurosci Lett* 187, 49-52.

Ahn A.C., Colbert A.P., Anderson B.J., Martinsen O.G., Hammerschlag R., Cina S., Wayne P.M., Langevin H.M., 2008. Electrical properties of acupuncture points and meridians: a systematic review. *Bioelectromagnetics* 29, 245-256.

Alimi D., Rubino C., Leandri E.P., Brule S.F., 2000. Analgesic effects of auricular acupuncture for cancer pain. *J Pain Symptom Manage* 19, 81-82.

Allen, J., Meires J., 2011. How to prescribe Tai chi therapy. *J Transcult Nurs* 22, 201-204.

Allman J.M., Hakeem A., Erwin J.M., Nimchinsky E., Hof P., 2001. The anterior cingulate cortex. The evolution of an interface between emotion and cognition. *Ann N Y Acad Sci* 935, 107-117.

Altman R.D., Marcussen K.C., 2001. Effects of a ginger extract on knee pain in patients with osteoarthritis. *Arthritis Rheum* 44, 2531-2538.

Amanzio M., Benedetti F., 1999. Neuropharmacological dissection of placebo analgesia: expectation-activated opioid systems versus conditioning-activated specific subsystems. J Neurosci 19, 484-494.

Andersson S., Lundeberg T., 1995. Acupuncture--from empiricism to science: functional background to acupuncture effects in pain and disease. *Med Hypotheses* 45, 271-281.

Angell M., 2004. Excess in the pharmaceutical industry. *CMAJ* 171, 1451-1453.

Angell M., 2009. Relationships with the drug industry: Keep at arm's length. *BMJ* 338, b222.

Arletti R., Bertolini A., 1987. Oxytocin acts as an antidepressant in two animal models of depression. *Life Sci* 41, 1725-1730.

Arnsten A.F., 2009. Stress signalling pathways that impair prefrontal cortex structure and function. *Nat Rev Neurosci* 10, 410-422.

Arthur H.M., Patterson C., Stone J.A., 2006. The role of complementary and alternative therapies in cardiac rehabilitation: a systematic evaluation. *Eur J Cardiovasc Prev Rehabil* 13, 3-9.

Ascherio A., 2002. Epidemiologic studies on dietary fats and coronary heart disease. *Am J Med* 113 Suppl 9B, 9S-12S.

Astin J.A., 1998. Why patients use alternative medicine: results of a national study. *Jama* 279, 1548-1553.

Attal N., Cruccu G., Baron R., Haanpaa M., Hansson P., Jensen T.S., Nurmikko T., 2010. EFNS guidelines on the pharmacological treatment of neuropathic pain: 2010 revision. *Eur J Neurol* 17, 1113-e1188.

Augustin P., Hains A.A., 1996. Effect of music on ambulatory surgery patients' preoperative anxiety. *AORN* J 63, 750, 753-758.

Babyak M., Blumenthal J.A., Herman S., Khatri P., Doraiswamy M., Moore K., Craighead W.E., Baldewicz T.T., Krishnan K.R., 2000. Exercise treatment for major depression: maintenance of therapeutic benefit at 10 months. *Psychosom Med* 62, 633-638.

Babygirija R., Cerjak D., Yoshimoto S., Gribovskaja-Rupp I., Bulbul M., Ludwig K., Takahashi T., 2012a. Affiliative behavior attenuates stress responses of GI tract via up-regulating hypothalamic oxytocin expression. *Auton Neurosci* 169, 28-33.

Babygirija R., Yoshimoto S., Gribovskaja-Rupp I., Bülbül M., Ludwig K., Takahashi T., 2012b. Social interaction attenuates stress responses following chronic stress in maternally separated rats. *Brain Res* 1469, 54-62.

Babygirija R., Zheng J., Bulbul M., Ludwig K., Takahashi T., 2010. Beneficial effects of social attachment to overcome daily stress. *Brain Res* 1352, 43-49.

Bachar E., 1998. Psychotherapy--an active agent: assessing the effectiveness of psychotherapy and its curative factors. *Isr J Psychiatry Relat Sci* 35, 128-135.

Bali B., Kovacs K.J., 2003. GABAergic control of neuropeptide gene expression in parvocellular neurons of the hypothalamic paraventricular nucleus. *Eur J Neurosci* 18, 1518-1526.

Bangalore N.G., Varambally S., 2012. Yoga therapy for Schizophrenia. *Int J Yoga* 5, 85-91.

Barbour L.A., McGuire D.B., Kirchhoff K.T., 1986. Nonanalgesic methods of pain control used by cancer outpatients. *Oncol Nurs Forum* 13, 56-60.

Barde Y.A., 1994. Neurotrophins: a family of proteins supporting the survival of neurons. *Prog Clin Biol Res* 390, 45-56.

Barnes P.M., Powell-Griner E., McFann K., Nahin R.L., 2004. Complementary and alternative medicine use among adults: United States, 2002. Adv Data, 1-19.

Baron Short E., Kose S., Mu Q., Borckardt J., Newberg A., George M.S., Kozel F.A., 2007. Regional brain activation during meditation shows time and practice effects: an exploratory FMRI study. *Evid Based Complement Alternat Med* 7, 121-127.

Barraza J.A., Zak P.J., 2009. Empathy toward strangers triggers oxytocin release and subsequent generosity. *Ann N Y Acad Sci* 1167, 182-189.

Bausell R.B., Lao L., Bergman S., Lee W.L., Berman B.M., 2005. Is acupuncture analgesia an expectancy effect? Preliminary evidence based on participants' perceived assignments in two placebo-controlled trials. *Eval Health Prof* 28, 9-26.

Bello D., White-Traut R., Schwertz D., Pournajafi-Nazarloo H., Carter C.S., 2008. An exploratory study of neurohormonal responses of healthy men to massage. *J Altern Complement Med* 14, 387-394.

Benedetti F., 1996. The opposite effects of the opiate antagonist naloxone and the cholecystokinin antagonist proglumide on placebo analgesia. Pain 64, 535-543.

Benjamin E.J., Larson M.G., Keyes M.J., Mitchell G.F., Vasan R.S., Keaney J.F., Jr., Lehman B.T., Fan S., Osypiuk E., Vita J.A., 2004. Clinical correlates and heritability of flow-mediated dilation in the community: the Framingham Heart Study. *Circulation* 109, 613-619.

Berkman L.F., Syme S.L., 1979. Social networks, host resistance, and mortality: a nine-year follow-up study of Alameda County residents. *Am J Epidemiol* 109, 186-204.

Birdee G.S., Wayne P.M., Davis R.B., Phillips R.S., Yeh G.Y., 2009. T'ai chi and qigong for health: patterns of use in the United States. *J Altern Complement Med* 15, 969-973.

Bittman B., Bruhn K.T., Stevens C., Westengard J., Umbach P.O., 2003. Recreational music-making: a cost-effective group interdisciplinary strategy for reducing burnout and improving mood states in long-term care workers. *Adv Mind Body Med* 19, 4-15.

Bittman B.B., Berk L.S., Felten D.L., Westengard J., Simonton O.C., Pappas J., Ninehouser M., 2001. Composite effects of group drumming music therapy on modulation of neuroendocrine-immune parameters in normal subjects. *Altern Ther Health Med* 7, 38-47.

Bittman B.B., Snyder C., Bruhn K.T., Liebfreid F., Stevens C.K., Westengard J., Umbach P.O., 2004. Recreational music-making: an integrative group intervention for reducing burnout and improving mood states in first year associate degree nursing students: insights and economic impact. *Int J Nurs Educ Scholarsh* 1, Article12.

Blair K., Geraci M., Devido J., McCaffrey D., Chen G., Vythilingam M., Ng P., Hollon N., Jones M., Blair R.J., Pine D.S., 2008. Neural response to self- and other referential praise and criticism in generalized social phobia. *Arch Gen Psychiatry* 65, 1176-1184.

Blancquaert J.P., Lefebvre R.A., Willems J.L., 1986. Emetic and antiemetic effects of opioids in the dog. *Eur J Pharmacol* 128, 143-150.

Blumenthal J.A., Sherwood A., Babyak M.A., Watkins L.L., Waugh R., Georgiades A., Bacon S.L., Hayano J., Coleman R.E., Hinderliter A., 2005. Effects of exercise and stress management training on markers of cardiovascular risk in patients with ischemic heart disease: a randomized controlled trial. *Jama* 293, 1626-1634.

Boecker H., Sprenger T., Spilker M.E., Henriksen G., Koppenhoefer M., Wagner K.J., Valet M., Berthele A., Tolle T.R., 2008. The runner's high: opioidergic mechanisms in the human brain. *Cereb Cortex* 18, 2523-2531.

Bolton M.M., Pittman A.J., Lo D.C., 2000. Brain-derived neurotrophic factor differentially regulates excitatory and inhibitory synaptic transmission in hippocampal cultures. *J Neurosci* 20, 3221-3232.

Booth F.W., Lees S.J., 2006. Physically active subjects should be the control group. *Med Sci Sports Exerc* 38, 405-406.

Bowman A.J., Clayton R.H., Murray A., Reed J.W., Subhan M.M., Ford G.A., 1997. Effects of aerobic exercise training and yoga on the baroreflex in healthy elderly persons. *Eur J Clin Invest* 27, 443-449.

Braquet P., Bourgain R.H., 1987. Anti-anaphylactic properties of BN 52021: a potent platelet activating factor antagonist. *Adv Exp Med Biol* 215, 215-235.

Breton J.D., Poisbeau P., Darbon P., 2009. Antinociceptive action of oxytocin involves inhibition of potassium channel currents in lamina II neurons of the rat spinal cord. *Mol Pain* 5, 63.

Broadwell S.D., Light K.C., 1999. Family support and cardiovascular responses in married couples during conflict and other interactions. *Int J Behav Med* 6, 40-63.

Brooker D.J., Snape M., Johnson E., Ward D., Payne M., 1997. Single case evaluation of the effects of aromatherapy and massage on disturbed behaviour in severe dementia. *Br J Clin Psychol* 36 (Pt 2), 287-296.

Brown S.L., Nesse R.M., Vinokur A.D., Smith D.M., 2003. Providing social support may be more beneficial than receiving it: results from a prospective study of mortality. *Psychol Sci* 14, 320-327.

Brugman T., Ferguson S., 2002. Physical exercise and improvements in mental health. *J Psychosoc Nurs Ment Health Serv* 40, 24-31.

Bryant R.A., Hung L., Guastella A.J., Mitchell P.B., 2012. Oxytocin as a moderator of hypnotizability. *Psychoneuroendocrinology* 37, 162-166.

Bulbul M., Babygirija R., Cerjak D., Yoshimoto S., Ludwig K., Takahashi T., 2011. Hypothalamic oxytocin attenuates CRF expression via GABA(A) receptors in rats. *Brain Res* 1387, 39-45.

Burri A., Heinrichs M., Schedlowski M., Kruger T.H., 2008. The acute effects of intranasal oxytocin administration on endocrine and sexual function in males. *Psychoneuroendocrinology* 33, 591-600.

Butt M.S., Sultan M.T., 2012. Ginger and its health claims: molecular aspects. *Crit Rev Food Sci Nutr* 51, 383-393.

Cade W.T., Reeds D.N., Mondy K.E., Overton E.T., Grassino J., Tucker S., Bopp C., Laciny E., Hubert S., Lassa-Claxton S., Yarasheski K.E., 2010. Yoga lifestyle intervention reduces blood pressure in HIV-infected adults with cardiovascular disease risk factors. *HIV Med* 11, 379-388.

Calvert E.L., Houghton L.A., Cooper P., Morris J., Whorwell P.J., 2002. Long-term improvement in functional dyspepsia using hypnotherapy. *Gastroenterology* 123, 1778-1785.

Camilleri M., Malagelada J.R., Kao P.C., Zinsmeister A.R., 1984. Effect of somatovisceral reflexes and selective dermatomal stimulation on postcibal antral pressure activity. *Am J Physiol* 247, G703-708.

Camilleri M., Mayer E.A., Drossman D.A., Heath A., Dukes G.E., McSorley D., Kong S., Mangel A.W., Northcutt A.R., 1999. Improvement in pain and bowel function in female irritable bowel patients with alosetron, a 5-HT3 receptor antagonist. *Aliment Pharmacol Ther* 13, 1149-1159.

Campbell E.G., Gruen R.L., Mountford J., Miller L.G., Cleary P.D., Blumenthal D., 2007. A national survey of physician-industry relationships. *N Engl J Med* 356, 1742-1750.

Campbell T.C., Parpia B., Chen J., 1998. Diet, lifestyle, and the etiology of coronary artery disease: the Cornell China study. *Am J Cardiol* 82, 18T-21T.

Carmichael M.S., Humbert R., Dixen J., Palmisano G., Greenleaf W., Davidson J.M., 1987. Plasma oxytocin increases in the human sexual response. *J Clin Endocrinol Metab* 64, 27-31.

Carmody J., Baer R.A., E L.B.L., Olendzki N., 2009. An empirical study of the mechanisms of mindfulness in a mindfulness-based stress reduction program. J Clin Psychol 65, 613-626.

Carpenter D.O., Briggs D.B., Strominger N., 1984. Peptide-induced emesis in dogs. *Behav Brain Res* 11, 277-281.

Carson J.W., Carson K.M., Porter L.S., Keefe F.J., Seewaldt V.L., 2009. Yoga of Awareness program for menopausal symptoms in breast cancer survivors: results from a randomized trial. *Support Care Cancer* 17, 1301-1309.

Carson J.W., Carson K.M., Porter L.S., Keefe F.J., Shaw H., Miller J.M., 2007. Yoga for women with metastatic breast cancer: results from a pilot study. *J Pain Symptom Manage* 33, 331-341.

Carson J.W., Keefe F.J., Lynch T.R., Carson K.M., Goli V., Fras A.M., Thorp S.R., 2005. Loving-kindness meditation for chronic low back pain: results from a pilot trial. *J Holist Nur*s 23, 287-304.

Carter C.S., 1992. Oxytocin and sexual behavior. *Neurosci Biobehav Rev* 16, 131-144.

Carter C.S., 1998. Neuroendocrine perspectives on social attachment and love. *Psychoneuroendocrinology* 23, 779-818.

Caspi O., Bell I.R., Rychener D., Gaudet T.W., Weil A.T., 2000. The Tower of Babel: communication and medicine: An essay on medical education and complementary-alternative medicine. *Arch Intern Med* 160, 3193-3195.

Cassel J., 1976. The contribution of the social environment to host resistance: the Fourth Wade Hampton Frost Lecture. *Am J Epidemiol* 104, 107-123.

Cassileth B.R., Vickers A.J., 2004. Massage therapy for symptom control: outcome study at a major cancer center. *J Pain Symptom Manage* 28, 244-249.

Cassileth B.R., Vickers A.J., Magill L.A., 2003. Music therapy for mood disturbance during hospitalization for autologous stem cell transplantation: a randomized controlled trial. *Cancer* 98, 2723-2729.

Cazalis M., Dayanithi G., Nordmann J.J., 1987a. Hormone release from isolated nerve endings of the rat neurohypophysis. *J Physiol* 390, 55-70.

Cazalis M., Dayanithi G., Nordmann J.J., 1987b. Requirements for hormone release from permeabilized nerve endings isolated from the rat neurohypophysis. *J Physiol* 390, 71-91.

Cerqueira J.J., Almeida O.F., Sousa N., 2008. The stressed prefrontal cortex. Left? Right! Brain Behav Immun 22, 630-638.

Chang C., 2012. Is Integrative Medicine the Next New Frontier in Medicine? *Clin Rev Allergy Immunol.*

Chang C.S., Ko C.W., Wu C.Y., Chen G.H., 2001. Effect of electrical stimulation on acupuncture points in diabetic patients with gastric dysrhythmia: a pilot study. *Digestion* 64, 184-190.

Chapell M.S., 1994. Inner speech and respiration: toward a possible mechanism of stress reduction. *Percept Mot Skills* 79, 803-811.

Chattha R., Nagarathna R., Padmalatha V., Nagendra H.R., 2008. Effect of yoga on cognitive functions in climacteric syndrome: a randomised control study. *Bjog* 115, 991-1000.

Chen J.D., Qian L., Ouyang H., Yin J., 2003. Gastric electrical stimulation with short pulses reduces vomiting but not dysrhythmias in dogs. *Gastroenterology* 124, 401-409.

Chen K.W., Berger C.C., Manheimer E., Forde D., Magidson J., Dachman L., Lejuez C.W., 2012a. Meditative therapies for reducing anxiety: a systematic review and meta-analysis of randomized controlled trials. *Depress Anxiety* 29, 545-562.

Chen M.L., Lin L.C., Wu S.C., Lin J.G., 1999. The effectiveness of acupressure in improving the quality of sleep of institutionalized residents. *J Gerontol A Biol Sci Med Sci* 54, M389-394.

Chen X.W., Sneed K.B., Zhou S.F., 2012b. Pharmacokinetic profiles of anticancer herbal medicines in humans and the clinical implications. *Curr Med Chem* 18, 3190-3210.

Cherkin D.C., Sherman K.J., Avins A.L., Erro J.H., Ichikawa L., Barlow W.E., Delaney K., Hawkes R., Hamilton L., Pressman A., Khalsa P.S., Deyo R.A., 2009. A randomized trial comparing acupuncture, simulated acupuncture, and usual care for chronic low back pain. *Arch Intern Med* 169, 858-866.

Chiesa A., 2009. Zen meditation: an integration of current evidence. *J Altern Complement Med* 15, 585-592.

Chiu Y.J., Chi A., Reid I.A., 1997. Cardiovascular and endocrine effects of acupuncture in hypertensive patients. *Clin Exp Hypertens* 19, 1047-1063.

Cho M.M., DeVries A.C., Williams J.R., Carter C.S., 1999. The effects of oxytocin and vasopressin on partner preferences in male and female prairie voles (Microtus ochrogaster). Behav Neurosci 113, 1071-1079.

Cholburi J., Hanucharurnkul S., Waikakul W., 2004. Effectsof music therapy on anxiety and pain in cancer patients. *Thai J Nurse Res* 8, 173–181.

Chou R., Huffman L.H., 2007. Nonpharmacologic therapies for acute and chronic low back pain: a review of the evidence for an American Pain Society/American College of Physicians clinical practice guideline. *Ann Intern Med* 147, 492-504.

Chu L.F., Angst M.S., Clark D., 2008. Opioid-induced hyperalgesia in humans: molecular mechanisms and clinical considerations. *Clin J Pain* 24, 479-496.

Clarkson P., Montgomery H.E., Mullen M.J., Donald A.E., Powe A.J., Bull T., Jubb M., World M., Deanfield J.E., 1999. Exercise training enhances endothelial function in young men. *J Am Coll Cardiol* 33, 1379-1385.

Coan J.A., Schaefer H.S., Davidson R.J., 2006. Lending a hand: social regulation of the neural response to threat. *Psychol Sci* 17, 1032-1039.

Cooke M., Chaboyer W., Schluter P., Hiratos M., 2005. The effect of music on preoperative anxiety in day surgery. *J Adv Nurs* 52, 47-55.

Corsetti M., Caenepeel P., Fischler B., Janssens J., Tack J., 2004. Impact of coexisting irritable bowel syndrome on symptoms and pathophysiological mechanisms in functional dyspepsia. *Am J Gastroenterol* 99, 1152-1159.

Costello D.J., Borison H.L., 1977. Naloxone antagonizes narcotic self blockade of emesis in the cat. J Pharmacol Exp Ther 203, 222-230.

Cottingham J.T., Porges S.W., Lyon T., 1988. Effects of soft tissue mobilization (Rolfing pelvic lift) on parasympathetic tone in two age groups. *Phys Ther* 68, 352-356.

Cowen V.S., 2010. Functional fitness improvements after a worksite-based yoga initiative. J Bodyw Mov Ther 14, 50-54.

Cowings P.S., Toscano W.B., 2000. Autogenic-feedback training exercise is superior to promethazine for control of motion sickness symptoms. *J Clin Pharmacol* 40, 1154-1165.

Craft T.K., Glasper E.R., McCullough L., Zhang N., Sugo N., Otsuka T., Hurn P.D., DeVries A.C., 2005. Social interaction improves experimental stroke outcome. *Stroke* 36, 2006-2011.

Cubeddu L.X., Lindley C.M., Wetsel W., Carl P.L., Negro-Vilar A., 1990. Role of angiotensin II and vasopressin in cisplatin-induced emesis. *Life Sci* 46, 699-705.

Cullinan W.E., 2000. GABA(A) receptor subunit expression within hypophysiotropic CRH neurons: a dual hybridization histochemical study. *J Comp Neurol* 419, 344-351.

Cullinan W.E., Ziegler D.R., Herman J.P., 2008. Functional role of local GABAergic influences on the HPA axis. *Brain Struct Funct* 213, 63-72.

Curtis D.R., Duggan A.W., Felix D., Johnston G.A., 1970. Bicuculline and central GABA receptors. *Nature* 228, 676-677.

Cyranowski J.M., Hofkens T.L., Frank E., Seltman H., Cai H.M., Amico J.A., 2008. Evidence of dysregulated peripheral oxytocin release among depressed women. *Psychosom Med* 70, 967-975.

Damodaran A., Malathi A., Patil N., Shah N., Suryavansihi, Marathe S., 2002. Therapeutic potential of yoga practices in modifying cardiovascular risk profile in middle aged men and women. *J Assoc Physicians India* 50, 633-640.

Danhauer S.C., Mihalko S.L., Russell G.B., Campbell C.R., Felder L., Daley K., Levine E.A., 2009. Restorative yoga for women with breast cancer: findings from a randomized pilot study. *Psychooncology* 18, 360-368.

Danhauer S.C., Tooze J.A., Farmer D.F., Campbell C.R., McQuellon R.P., Barrett R., Miller B.E., 2008. Restorative yoga for women with ovarian or breast cancer: findings from a pilot study. *J Soc Integr Oncol* 6, 47-58.

Davidson L., Haglund K.E., Stayner D.A., Rakfeldt J., Chinman M.J., Tebes J.K., 2001a. "It was just realizing ... that life isn't one big horror": a qualitative study of supported socialization. *Psychiatr Rehabil* J 24, 275-292.

Davidson L., Stayner D.A., Nickou C., Styron T.H., Rowe M., Chinman M.L., 2001b. "Simply to be let in": inclusion as a basis for recovery. *Psychiatr Rehabil J* 24, 375-388.

Davis E.L., Oh B., Butow P.N., Mullan B.A., Clarke S., 2012. Cancer patient disclosure and patient-doctor communication of complementary and alternative medicine use: a systematic review. *Oncologist* 17, 1475-1481.

de la Fuente-Fernandez R., Schulzer M., Stoessl A.J., 2004. Placebo mechanisms and reward circuitry: clues from Parkinson's disease. *Biol Psychiatry* 56, 67-71.

DeKosky S.T., Williamson J.D., Fitzpatrick A.L., Kronmal R.A., Ives D.G., Saxton J.A., Lopez O.L., Burke G., Carlson M.C., Fried L.P., Kuller L.H., Robbins J.A., Tracy R.P., Woolard N.F., Dunn L., Snitz B.E., Nahin R.L., Furberg C.D., 2008. Ginkgo biloba for prevention of dementia: a randomized controlled trial. *Jama* 300, 2253-2262.

Deng G., Cassileth B.R., 2005. Integrative oncology: complementary therapies for pain, anxiety, and mood disturbance. *CA Cancer J Clin* 55, 109-116.

Deng G.E., Cassileth B.R., Cohen L., Gubili J., Johnstone P.A., Kumar N., Vickers A., Abrams D., Rosenthal D., Sagar S., Tripathy D., 2007. Integrative Oncology Practice Guidelines. *J Soc Integr Oncol* 5, 65-84.

Detillion C.E., Craft T.K., Glasper E.R., Prendergast B.J., DeVries A.C., 2004. Social facilitation of wound healing. *Psychoneuroendocrinology* 29, 1004-1011.

DeVries A.C., Glasper E.R., Detillion C.E., 2003. Social modulation of stress responses. *Physiol Behav* 79, 399-407.

Di S., Tasker J.G., 2008. Rapid synapse-specific regulation of hypothalamic magnocellular neurons by glucocorticoids. *Prog Brain Res* 170, 379-388.

Diehl D.L., 1999. Acupuncture for gastrointestinal and hepatobiliary disorders. *J Altern Complement Med* 5, 27-45.

Ditzen B., Schaer M., Gabriel B., Bodenmann G., Ehlert U., Heinrichs M., 2009. Intranasal oxytocin increases positive communication and reduces cortisol levels during couple conflict. *Biol Psychiatry* 65, 728-731.

Dobos G.J., Kirschbaum B., Choi K.E., 2012. The Western model of integrative oncology: the contribution of Chinese medicine. *Chin J Integr Med* 18, 643-651.

Dodge H.H., Zitzelberger T., Oken B.S., Howieson D., Kaye J., 2008. A randomized placebo-controlled trial of Ginkgo biloba for the prevention of cognitive decline. *Neurology* 70, 1809-1817.

Dovidio j., Piliavin J., Schroeder D., Penner L., 2006. The social psychology of personal behavior. Psychology Press, New York.

Drossman D.A., 2006. The functional gastrointestinal disorders and the Rome III process. *Gastroenterology* 130, 1377-1390.

Droste S.K., Chandramohan Y., Hill L.E., Linthorst A.C., Reul J.M., 2007. Voluntary exercise impacts on the rat hypothalamic-pituitary-adrenocortical axis mainly at the adrenal level. *Neuroendocrinology* 86, 26-37.

Dunbar R.I., 2010. The social role of touch in humans and primates: behavioural function and neurobiological mechanisms. *Neurosci Biobehav Rev* 34, 260-268.

Duncan M.D., Leis A., Taylor-Brown J.W., 2008. Impact and outcomes of an Iyengar yoga program in a cancer centre. *Curr Oncol* 15 Suppl 2, s109 es172-108.

Dundee J., Ghaly R., Fitzpatrick K., al e., 1987. Acupuncture to prevent cisplatin-associated vomiting. *Lancet* 1, 1083.

Dundee J.W., Ghaly R.G., Bill K.M., Chestnutt W.N., Fitzpatrick K.T., Lynas A.G., 1989. Effect of stimulation of the P6 antiemetic point on postoperative nausea and vomiting. *Br J Anaesth* 63, 612-618.

Dusseldorp E., van Elderen T., Maes S., Meulman J., Kraaij V., 1999. A meta-analysis of psychoeduational programs for coronary heart disease patients. *Health Psychol* 18, 506-519.

Dworkin B.R., Elbert T., Rau H., Birbaumer N., Pauli P., Droste C., Brunia C.H., 1994. Central effects of baroreceptor activation in humans: attenuation of skeletal reflexes and pain perception. *Proc Natl Acad Sci U S A* 91, 6329-6333.

Edwards C.M., Carmichael J., Baylis P.H., Harris A.L., 1989. Arginine vasopressin--a mediator of chemotherapy induced emesis? *Br J Cancer* 59, 467-470.

Egan M.F., Weinberger D.R., Lu B., 2003. Schizophrenia, III: brain-derived neurotropic factor and genetic risk. *Am J Psychiatry* 160, 1242.

Eisenberg D.M., 1997. Advising patients who seek alternative medical therapies. *Ann Intern Med* 127, 61-69.

Eisenberg D.M., Davis R.B., Ettner S.L., Appel S., Wilkey S., Van Rompay M., Kessler R.C., 1998. Trends in alternative medicine use in the United States, 1990-1997: results of a follow-up national survey. *Jama* 280, 1569-1575.

Ekkekakis P., Hall E.E., VanLanduyt L.M., Petruzzello S.J., 2000. Walking in (affective) circles: can short walks enhance affect? *J Behav Med* 23, 245-275.

Elkin I., Shea M.T., Watkins J.T., Imber S.D., Sotsky S.M., Collins J.F., Glass D.R., Pilkonis P.A., Leber W.R., Docherty J.P., et al., 1989. National Institute of Mental Health Treatment of Depression Collaborative Research Program. General effectiveness of treatments. *Arch Gen Psychiatry* 46, 971-982; discussion 983.

Elkins G., Fisher W., Johnson A., 2010. Mind-body therapies in integrative oncology. *Curr Treat Options Oncol* 11, 128-140.

Elkins G., Jensen M.P., Patterson D.R., 2007. Hypnotherapy for the management of chronic pain. *Int J Clin Exp Hypn* 55, 275-287.

Enck P., Benedetti F., Schedlowski M., 2008. New insights into the placebo and nocebo responses. *Neuron* 59, 195-206.

Enck P., Klosterhalfen S., 2009. The story of O--is oxytocin the mediator of the placebo response? *Neurogastroenterol Motil* 21, 347-350.

Erickson K.I., Voss M.W., Prakash R.S., Basak C., Szabo A., Chaddock L., Kim J.S., Heo S., Alves H., White S.M., Wojcicki T.R., Mailey E., Vieira V.J., Martin S.A., Pence B.D., Woods J.A., McAuley E., Kramer A.F., 2011. Exercise training increases size of hippocampus and improves memory. *Proc Natl Acad Sci U S A* 108, 3017-3022.

Ernst E., Kanji N., 2000. Autogenic training for stress and anxiety: a systematic review. Complement Ther Med 8, 106-110.

Esch T., Stefano G.B., 2005. The Neurobiology of Love. *Neuro Endocrinol Lett* 26, 175-192.

Evans S., Moieni M., Taub R., Subramanian S.K., Tsao J.C., Sternlieb B., Zeltzer L.K., 2010. Iyengar yoga for young adults with rheumatoid arthritis: results from a mixed-methods pilot study. *J Pain Symptom Manage 3*9, 904-913.

Ezzo J., Berman B., Hadhazy V.A., Jadad A.R., Lao L., Singh B.B., 2000. Is acupuncture effective for the treatment of chronic pain? A systematic review. *Pain* 86, 217-225.

Falkenberg T., Mohammed A.K., Henriksson B., Persson H., Winblad B., Lindefors N., 1992. Increased expression of brain-derived neurotrophic factor mRNA in rat hippocampus is associated with improved spatial memory and enriched environment. *Neurosci Lett* 138, 153-156.

Farb N.A., Segal Z.V., Anderson A.K., 2012. Mindfulness meditation training alters cortical representations of interoceptive attention. Soc Cogn Affect Neurosci.

Farb N.A., Segal Z.V., Mayberg H., Bean J., McKeon D., Fatima Z., Anderson A.K., 2007. Attending to the present: mindfulness meditation reveals distinct neural modes of self-reference. *Soc Cogn Affect Neurosci* 2, 313-322.

Feldman R., Gordon I., Zagoory-Sharon O., 2010. Maternal and paternal plasma, salivary, and urinary oxytocin and parent-infant synchrony: considering stress and affiliation components of human bonding. *Dev Sci* 14, 752-761.

Ferguson J.N., Young L.J., Hearn E.F., Matzuk M.M., Insel T.R., Winslow J.T., 2000. Social amnesia in mice lacking the oxytocin gene. *Nat Genet* 25, 284-288.

Ferrell-Torry A.T., Glick O.J., 1993. The use of therapeutic massage as a nursing intervention to modify anxiety and the perception of cancer pain. *Cancer Nurs* 16, 93-101.

Field T., 2002. Massage therapy. *Med Clin North Am* 86, 163-171.

Field T., 2011. Yoga clinical research review. *Complement Ther Clin Pract* 17, 1-8.

Field T., Morrow C., Valdeon C., Larson S., Kuhn C., Schanberg S., 1992. Massage reduces anxiety in child and adolescent psychiatric patients. *J Am Acad Child Adolesc Psychiatry* 31, 125-131.

Field T., Peck M., Krugman S., Tuchel T., Schanberg S., Kuhn C., Burman I., 1998. Burn injuries benefit from massage therapy. *J Burn Care Rehabil* 19, 241-244.

Field T.M., 1998. Massage therapy effects. *Am Psychol* 53, 1270-1281.

Filippi S., Vignozzi L., Vannelli G.B., Ledda F., Forti G., Maggi M., 2003. Role of oxytocin in the ejaculatory process. *J Endocrinol Invest* 26, 82-86.

Fisher P., McCarney R., Hasford C., Vickers A., 2006. Evaluation of specific and non-specific effects in homeopathy: feasibility study for a randomised trial. *Homeopathy* 95, 215-222.

Fisher P., Ward A., 1994. Complementary medicine in Europe. *Bmj* 309, 107-111.

Flachskampf F.A., Gallasch J., Gefeller O., Gan J., Mao J., Pfahlberg A.B., Wortmann A., Klinghammer L., Pflederer W., Daniel W.G., 2007. Randomized trial of acupuncture to lower blood pressure. *Circulation* 115, 3121-3129.

Fleming I., Busse R., 2003. Molecular mechanisms involved in the regulation of the endothelial nitric oxide synthase. *Am J Physiol Regul Integr Comp Physiol* 284, R1-12.

Fleming S., Rabago D.P., Mundt M.P., Fleming M.F., 2007. CAM therapies among primary care patients using opioid therapy for chronic pain. *BMC Complement Altern Med* 7, 15.

Flor H., Braun C., Elbert T., Birbaumer N., 1997. Extensive reorganization of primary somatosensory cortex in chronic back pain patients. *Neurosci Lett* 224, 5-8.

Flor H., Denke C., Schaefer M., Grusser S., 2001. Effect of sensory discrimination training on cortical reorganisation and phantom limb pain. *Lancet* 357, 1763-1764.

Foley E., Baillie A., Huxter M., Price M., Sinclair E., 2010. Mindfulness-based cognitive therapy for individuals whose lives have been affected by cancer: a randomized controlled trial. *J Consult Clin Psychol* 78, 72-79.

Fonberg E., Kostarczyk E., Prechtl J., 1981. Training of instrumental responses in dogs socially reinforced by humans. *Pavlov J Biol Sci* 16, 183-193.

Foss J.F., Yuan C.S., Roizen M.F., Goldberg L.I., 1998. Prevention of apomorphine- or cisplatin-induced emesis in the dog by a combination of methylnaltrexone and morphine. Cancer Chemother Pharmacol 42, 287-291.

Fournier J.C., DeRubeis R.J., Hollon S.D., Dimidjian S., Amsterdam J.D., Shelton R.C., Fawcett J., 2010. Antidepressant drug effects and depression severity: a patient-level meta-analysis. *Jama* 303, 47-53.

Francis S., Rolls E.T., Bowtell R., McGlone F., O'Doherty J., Browning A., Clare S., Smith E., 1999. The representation of pleasant touch in the brain and its relationship with taste and olfactory areas. *Neuroreport* 10, 453-459.

Fransen M., McConnell S., 2009a. Land-based exercise for osteoarthritis of the knee: a metaanalysis of randomized controlled trials. *J Rheumatol* 36, 1109-1117.

Fransen M., McConnell S., Hernandez-Molina G., Reichenbach S., 2009b. Exercise for osteoarthritis of the hip. *Cochrane Database Syst Rev,* CD007912.

Frasch A., Zetzsche T., Steiger A., Jirikowski G.F., 1995. Reduction of plasma oxytocin levels in patients suffering from major depression. *Adv Exp Med Biol* 395, 257-258.

Frass M., Strassl R.P., Friehs H., Mullner M., Kundi M., Kaye A.D., 2012. Use and acceptance of complementary and alternative medicine among the general population and medical personnel: a systematic review. *Ochsner* J 12, 45-56.

Frasure-Smith N., Lesperance F., Talajic M., 1995a. Depression and 18-month prognosis after myocardial infarction. *Circulation* 91, 999-1005.

Frasure-Smith N., Lesperance F., Talajic M., 1995b. The impact of negative emotions on prognosis following myocardial infarction: is it more than depression? *Health Psychol* 14, 388-398.

Fredrickson B.L., Cohn M.A., Coffey K.A., Pek J., Finkel S.M., 2008. Open hearts build lives: positive emotions, induced through loving-kindness meditation, build consequential personal resources. *J Pers Soc Psychol* 95, 1045-1062.

Fricchione G., Stefano G.B., 2005. Placebo neural systems: nitric oxide, morphine and the dopamine brain reward and motivation circuitries. *Med Sci Monit* 11, MS54-65.

Fridovich I., 1999. Fundamental aspects of reactive oxygen species, or what's the matter with oxygen? *Ann N Y Acad Sci* 893, 13-18.

Froeliger B.E., Garland E.L., Modlin L.A., McClernon F.J., 2012. Neurocognitive correlates of the effects of yoga meditation practice on emotion and cognition: a pilot study. Front Integr Neurosci 6, 48.

Fukai T., Siegfried M.R., Ushio-Fukai M., Cheng Y., Kojda G., Harrison D.G., 2000. Regulation of the vascular extracellular superoxide dismutase by nitric oxide and exercise training. *J Clin Invest* 105, 1631-1639.

Fukui H., Yamashita M., 2003. The effects of music and visual stress on testosterone and cortisol in men and women. *Neuro Endocrinol Lett* 24, 173-180.

Fukumoto S., Tatewaki M., Yamada T., Fujimiya M., Mantyh C., Voss M., Eubanks S., Harris M., Pappas T.N., Takahashi T., 2003. Short-chain fatty acids stimulate colonic transit via intraluminal 5-HT release in rats. *Am J Physiol Regul Integr Comp Physiol* 284, R1269-1276.

Funk J.L., Frye J.B., Oyarzo J.N., Kuscuoglu N., Wilson J., McCaffrey G., Stafford G., Chen G., Lantz R.C., Jolad S.D., Solyom A.M., Kiela P.R., Timmermann B.N., 2006. Efficacy and mechanism of action of turmeric supplements in the treatment of experimental arthritis. *Arthritis Rheum* 54, 3452-3464.

Furlan A.D., Sandoval J.A., Mailis-Gagnon A., Tunks E., 2006. Opioids for chronic noncancer pain: a meta-analysis of effectiveness and side effects. *Cmaj* 174, 1589-1594.

Furlan A.D., Yazdi F., Tsertsvadze A., Gross A., Van Tulder M., Santaguida L., Gagnier J., Ammendolia C., Dryden T., Doucette S., Skidmore B., Daniel R., Ostermann T., Tsouros S., A systematic review and meta-analysis of efficacy, cost-effectiveness, and safety of selected complementary and alternative medicine for neck and low-back pain. *Evid Based Complement Alternat Med* 2012, 953139.

Gaman A., Bucur M.C., Kuo B., 2009. Therapeutic advances in functional gastrointestinal disease: irritable bowel syndrome. *Therap Adv Gastroenterol* 2, 169-181.

Gamboa-Esteves F.O., Lima D., Batten T.F., 2001. Neurochemistry of superficial spinal neurones projecting to nucleus of the solitary tract that express c-fos on chemical somatic and visceral nociceptive input in the rat. *Metab Brain Dis* 16, 151-164.

Gan T.J., Jiao K.R., Zenn M., Georgiade G., 2004. A randomized controlled comparison of electro-acupoint stimulation or ondansetron versus placebo for the prevention of postoperative nausea and vomiting. Anesth Analg 99, 1070-1075, table of contents.

Gao M., Wang M., Li K., He L., 1997. Changes of mu opioid receptor binding sites in rat brain following electroacupuncture. *Acupunct Electrother Res* 22, 161-166.

Garfinkel M.S., Schumacher H.R., Jr., Husain A., Levy M., Reshetar R.A., 1994. Evaluation of a yoga based regimen for treatment of osteoarthritis of the hands. *J Rheumatol* 21, 2341-2343.

Garland E.L., Gaylord S.A., Palsson O., Faurot K., Douglas Mann J., Whitehead W.E., 2011. Therapeutic mechanisms of a mindfulness-based treatment for IBS: effects on visceral sensitivity, catastroph*izing, and affective processing of pain sensations.* J Behav Med.

Gaylord S.A., Palsson O.S., Garland E.L., Faurot K.R., Coble R.S., Mann J.D., Frey W., Leniek K., Whitehead W.E., 2011. Mindfulness training reduces the severity of irritable bowel syndrome in women: results of a randomized controlled trial. *Am J Gastroenterol* 106, 1678-1688.

Ghione S., 1996. Hypertension-associated hypalgesia. Evidence in experimental animals and humans, pathophysiological mechanisms, and potential clinical consequences. *Hypertension* 28, 494-504.

Gielen S., Erbs S., Linke A., Mobius-Winkler S., Schuler G., Hambrecht R., 2003. Home-based versus hospital-based exercise programs in patients with coronary artery disease: effects on coronary vasomotion. *Am Heart J* 145, E3.

Glasper E.R., Devries A.C., 2005. Social structure influences effects of pair-housing on wound healing. *Brain Behav Immun* 19, 61-68.

Gokal R., Shillito L., Maharaj S.R., 2007. Positive impact of yoga and pranayam on obesity, hypertension, blood sugar, and cholesterol: a pilot assessment. *J Altern Complement Med* 13, 1056-1057.

Golbidi S., Laher I., 2012. Exercise and the cardiovascular system. *Cardiol Res Pract* 2012, 210852.

Goldin P.R., Gross J.J., 2010. Effects of mindfulness-based stress reduction (MBSR) on emotion regulation in social anxiety disorder. *Emotion* 10, 83-91.

Gomez-Cabrera M.C., Domenech E., Vina J., 2008. Moderate exercise is an antioxidant: upregulation of antioxidant genes by training. F*ree Radic Biol Med* 44, 126-131.

Gonzaga G.C., Turner R.A., Keltner D., Campos B., Altemus M., 2006. Romantic love and sexual desire in close relationships. *Emotion* 6, 163-179.

Good M., Stanton-Hicks M., Grass J.A., Cranston Anderson G., Choi C., Schoolmeesters L.J., Salman A., 1999. Relief of postoperative pain with jaw relaxation, music and their combination. *Pain* 81, 163-172.

Grape C., Sandgren M., Hansson L.O., Ericson M., Theorell T., 2003. Does singing promote well-being?: An empirical study of professional and amateur singers during a singing lesson. *Integr Physiol Behav Sci* 38, 65-74.

Grewen K.M., Anderson B.J., Girdler S.S., Light K.C., 2003. Warm partner contact is related to lower cardiovascular reactivity. *Behav Med* 29, 123-130.

Grewen K.M., Girdler S.S., Amico J., Light K.C., 2005. Effects of partner support on resting oxytocin, cortisol, norepinephrine, and blood pressure before and after warm partner contact. *Psychosom Med* 67, 531-538.

Grewen K.M., Light K.C., Mechlin B., Girdler S.S., 2008. Ethnicity is associated with alterations in oxytocin relationships to pain sensitivity in women. *Ethn Health* 13, 219-241.

Griffin M.R., Scheiman J.M., 2001. Prospects for changing the burden of nonsteroidal anti-inflammatory drug toxicity. *Am J Med* 110, 33S-37S.

Grippo A.J., Gerena D., Huang J., Kumar N., Shah M., Ughreja R., Carter C.S., 2007. Social isolation induces behavioral and neuroendocrine disturbances relevant to depression in female and male prairie voles. *Psychoneuroendocrinology* 32, 966-980.

Grodin M.A., Piwowarczyk L., Fulker D., Bazazi A.R., Saper R.B., 2008. Treating survivors of torture and refugee trauma: a preliminary case series using qigong and t'ai chi. *J Altern Complement Med* 14, 801-806.

Grossman A., Bouloux P., Price P., Drury P.L., Lam K.S., Turner T., Thomas J., Besser G.M., Sutton J., 1984. The role of opioid peptides in the hormonal responses to acute exercise in man. *Clin Sci (Lond)* 67, 483-491.

Grossman P., Niemann L., Schmidt S., Walach H., 2004. Mindfulness-based stress reduction and health benefits. A meta-analysis. *J Psychosom Res* 57, 35-43.

Guarneri M., Mercado N., Suhar C., 2009. Integrative approaches for cardiovascular disease. *Nutr Clin Pract* 24, 701-708.

Guggenheimer J., Moore P.A., 2011. The therapeutic applications of and risks associated with acetaminophen use: a review and update. *J Am Dent Assoc* 142, 38-44.

Guo H.F., Wang X.M., Tian J.H., Huo Y.P., Han J.S., 1997. 2 Hz and 100 Hz electroacupuncture accelerate the expression of genes encoding three opioid peptides in the rat brain. *Sheng Li Xue Bao* 49, 121-127.

Guo Z.L., Longhurst J.C., 2007. Expression of c-Fos in arcuate nucleus induced by electroacupuncture: relations to neurons containing opioids and glutamate. *Brain R*es 1166, 65-76.

Guo Z.L., Moazzami A.R., Longhurst J.C., 2004. Electroacupuncture induces c-Fos expression in the rostral ventrolateral medulla and periaqueductal gray in cats: relation to opioid containing neurons. *Brain Res* 1030, 103-115.

Gutkowska J., Jankowski M., 2012. Oxytocin revisited: its role in cardiovascular regulation. *J Neuroendocrinol* 24, 599-608.

Gutkowska J., Jankowski M., Mukaddam-Daher S., McCann S.M., 2000. Oxytocin is a cardiovascular hormone. *Braz J Med Biol Res* 33, 625-633.

Hallstrom C., 1982. Effect of ginseng on the performance of nurses on night duty. *Comp Med East West* 6, 277–282.

Hambrecht R., Adams V., Erbs S., Linke A., Krankel N., Shu Y., Baither Y., Gielen S., Thiele H., Gummert J.F., Mohr F.W., Schuler G., 2003. Regular physical activity improves endothelial function in patients with coronary artery disease by increasing phosphorylation of endothelial nitric oxide synthase. *Circulation* 107, 3152-3158.

Hambrecht R., Fiehn E., Weigl C., Gielen S., Hamann C., Kaiser R., Yu J., Adams V., Niebauer J., Schuler G., 1998. Regular physical exercise corrects endothelial dysfunction and improves exercise capacity in patients with chronic heart failure. *Circulation* 98, 2709-2715.

Hambrecht R., Walther C., Mobius-Winkler S., Gielen S., Linke A., Conradi K., Erbs S., Kluge R., Kendziorra K., Sabri O., Sick P., Schuler G., 2004. Percutaneous coronary angioplasty compared with exercise training in patients with stable coronary artery disease: a randomized trial. *Circulation* 109, 1371-1378.

Hammar M., Frisk J., Grimas O., Hook M., Spetz A.C., Wyon Y., 1999. Acupuncture treatment of vasomotor symptoms in men with prostatic carcinoma: a pilot study. *J Urol* 161, 853-856.

Hampton A.N., O'Doherty J P., 2007. Decoding the neural substrates of reward-related decision making with functional MRI. *Proc Natl Acad Sci U S A* 104, 1377-1382.

Han S.H., Yoon S.H., Cho Y.W., Kim C.J., Min B.I., 1999. Inhibitory effects of electroacupuncture on stress responses evoked by tooth-pulp stimulation in rats. *Physiol Beha*v 66, 217-222.

Hanai F., 2000. Effect of electrical stimulation of peripheral nerves on neuropathic pain. *Spine* (Phila Pa 1976) 25, 1886-1892.

Harber V.J., Sutton J.R., 1984. Endorphins and exercise. *Sports Med* 1, 154-171.

Harburg E., Blakelock E.H., Jr., Roeper P.R., 1979. Resentful and reflective coping with arbitrary authority and blood pressure: *Detroit. Psychosom Med* 41, 189-202.

Hariri A.R., Goldberg T.E., Mattay V.S., Kolachana B.S., Callicott J.H., Egan M.F., Weinberger D.R., 2003. Brain-derived neurotrophic factor val66met polymorphism affects human memory-related hippocampal activity and predicts memory performance. *J Neurosci* 23, 6690-6694.

Hart C.E., Tracy B.L., 2008. Yoga as steadiness training: effects on motor variability in young adults. *J Strength Cond Res* 22, 1659-1669.

Hawkley L.C., Masi C.M., Berry J.D., Cacioppo J.T., 2006. Loneliness is a unique predictor of age-related differences in systolic blood pressure. *Psychol Aging* 21, 152-164.

Heinrichs M., Baumgartner T., Kirschbaum C., Ehlert U., 2003. Social support and oxytocin interact to suppress cortisol and subjective responses to psychosocial stress. *Biol Psychiatry* 54, 1389-1398.

Helms J.M., 1998. An overview of medical acupuncture. *Altern Ther Health Med* 4, 35-45.

Hendelman W., Humphreys P., Skinner C., 2010. The integrated nervous sytem. CRC press, Boca Raton, FL.

Hermann R., von Richter O., 2012. Clinical evidence of herbal drugs as perpetrators of pharmacokinetic drug interactions. *Planta Med* 78, 1458-1477.

Hernandez H., Serafin N., Terrazas A.M., Marnet P.G., Kann G., Delgadillo J.A., Poindron P., 2002. Maternal olfaction differentially modulates oxytocin and prolactin release during suckling in goats. *Horm Behav* 42, 232-244.

Hernandez-Reif M., Martinez A., Field T., Quintero O., Hart S., Burman I., 2000. Premenstrual symptoms are relieved by massage therapy. *J Psychosom Obstet Gynaecol* 21, 9-15.

Higashi Y., Sasaki S., Kurisu S., Yoshimizu A., Sasaki N., Matsuura H., Kajiyama G., Oshima T., 1999. Regular aerobic exercise augments endothelium-dependent vascular relaxation in normotensive as well as hypertensive subjects: role of endothelium-derived nitric oxide. *Circulation* 100, 1194-1202.

Hillman C.H., Erickson K.I., Kramer A.F., 2008. Be smart, exercise your heart: exercise effects on brain and cognition. *Nat Rev Neurosci* 9, 58-65.

Hirschfeld R.M., Montgomery S.A., Aguglia E., Amore M., Delgado P.L., Gastpar M., Hawley C., Kasper S., Linden M., Massana J., Mendlewicz J., Moller H.J., Nemeroff C.B., Saiz J., Such P., Torta R., Versiani M., 2002. Partial response and nonresponse to antidepressant therapy: current approaches and treatment options. *J Clin Psychiatry* 63, 826-837.

Ho P., Tsao J.C., Bloch L., Zeltzer L.K., 2011. The impact of group drumming on social-emotional behavior in low-income children. *Evid Based Complement Alternat Med* 2011, 250708.

Hollifield M., Sinclair-Lian N., Warner T.D., Hammerschlag R., 2007. Acupuncture for posttraumatic stress disorder: a randomized controlled pilot trial. *J Nerv Ment Dis* 195, 504-513.

Holmes M.D., Chen W.Y., Feskanich D., Kroenke C.H., Colditz G.A., 2005. Physical activity and survival after breast cancer diagnosis. *Jama* 293, 2479-2486.

Holst S., Uvnas-Moberg K., Petersson M., 2002. Postnatal oxytocin treatment and postnatal stroking of rats reduce blood pressure in adulthood. *Auton Neurosci* 99, 85-90.

Holzel B.K., Carmody J., Vangel M., Congleton C., Yerramsetti S.M., Gard T., Lazar S.W., 2011. Mindfulness practice leads to increases in regional brain gray matter density. *Psychiatry Res* 191, 36-43.

Hong C.Z., 1994. Lidocaine injection versus dry needling to myofascial trigger point. The importance of the local twitch response. *Am J Phys Med Rehabil* 73, 256-263.

House J.S., Landis K.R., Umberson D., 1988. Social relationships and health. *Science* 241, 540-545.

House J.S., Robbins C., Metzner H.L., 1982. The association of social relationships and activities with mortality: prospective evidence from the Tecumseh Community Health Study. *Am J Epidemiol* 116, 123-140.

Hu F.B., Stampfer M.J., Manson J.E., Rimm E., Colditz G.A., Rosner B.A., Hennekens C.H., Willett W.C., 1997. Dietary fat intake and the risk of coronary heart disease in women. *N Engl J Med* 337, 1491-1499.

Hu S., Stern R.M., Koch K.L., 1992. Electrical acustimulation relieves vection-induced motion sickness. *Gastroenterology* 102, 1854-1858.

Huber D., Veinante P., Stoop R., 2005. Vasopressin and oxytocin excite distinct neuronal populations in the central amygdala. *Science* 308, 245-248.

Hulme J., Waterman H., Hillier V.F., 1999. The effect of foot massage on patients' perception of care following laparoscopic sterilization as day case patients. *J Adv Nurs* 30, 460-468.

Hutcherson C.A., Seppala E.M., Gross J.J., 2008. Loving-kindness meditation increases social connectedness. *Emotion* 8, 720-724.

Imai K., Ariga H., Chen C., Mantyh C., Pappas T.N., Takahashi T., 2008. Effects of electroacupuncture on gastric motility and heart rate variability in conscious rats. *Auton Neurosci* 138, 91-98.

Imai K., Ariga H., Takahashi T., 2009. Electroacupuncture improves imbalance of autonomic function under restraint stress in conscious rats. *Am J Chin Med* 37, 45-55.

Inenaga K., Yamashita H., 1986. Excitation of neurones in the rat paraventricular nucleus in vitro by vasopressin and oxytocin. *J Physiol* 370, 165-180.

Innes K.E., Bourguignon C., Taylor A.G., 2005. Risk indices associated with the insulin resistance syndrome, cardiovascular disease, and possible protection with yoga: a systematic review. *J Am Board Fam Pract* 18, 491-519.

Ironson G., Field T., Scafidi F., Hashimoto M., Kumar M., Kumar A., Price A., Goncalves A., Burman I., Tetenman C., Patarca R., Fletcher M.A., 1996. Massage therapy is associated with enhancement of the immune system's cytotoxic capacity. *Int J Neurosci* 84, 205-217.

Ishak W.W., Berman D.S., Peters A., 2008. Male anorgasmia treated with oxytocin. *J Sex Med* 5, 1022-1024.

Itoh K., Asai S., Ohyabu H., Imai K., Kitakoji H., 2012. Effects of trigger point acupuncture treatment on temporomandibular disorders: a preliminary randomized clinical trial. *J Acupunct Meridian Stud* 5, 57-62.

Itoh K., Katsumi Y., Hirota S., Kitakoji H., 2007. Randomised trial of trigger point acupuncture compared with other acupuncture for treatment of chronic neck pain. *Complement Ther Med* 15, 172-179.

Itoh K., Katsumi Y., Kitakoji H., 2004. Trigger point acupuncture treatment of chronic low back pain in elderly patients--a blinded RCT. *Acupunct Med* 22, 170-177.

Itoh T., Yamakawa J., Mai M., Yamaguchi N., Kanda T., 2002. The effect of the herbal medicine dai-kenchu-to on post-operative ileus. *J Int Med Res* 30, 428-432.

Iwa M., Nakade Y., Pappas T.N., Takahashi T., 2006. Electroacupuncture elicits dual effects: stimulation of delayed gastric emptying and inhibition of accelerated colonic transit induced by restraint stress in rats. *Dig Dis Sci* 51, 1493-1500.

Iwa M., Strickland C., Nakade Y., Pappas T.N., Takahashi T., 2005. Electroacupuncture reduces rectal distension-induced blood pressure changes in conscious dogs. *Dig Dis Sci* 50, 1264-1270.

Iwa M., Tateiwa M., Sakita M., Fujimiya M., Takahashi T., 2007. Anatomical evidence of regional specific effects of acupuncture on gastric motor function in rats. *Auton Neurosci* 137, 67-76.

Jacobs B.L., Fornal C.A., 1993. 5-HT and motor control: a hypothesis. *Trends Neurosci* 16, 346-352.

Janal M.N., Colt E.W., Clark W.C., Glusman M., 1984. Pain sensitivity, mood and plasma endocrine levels in man following long-distance running: effects of naloxone. *Pain* 19, 13-25.

Jankowski M., Wang D., Hajjar F., Mukaddam-Daher S., McCann S.M., Gutkowska J., 2000. Oxytocin and its receptors are synthesized in the rat vasculature. *Proc Natl Acad Sci U S A* 97, 6207-6211.

Jansen M.J., Viechtbauer W., Lenssen A.F., Hendriks E.J., de Bie R.A., 2011. Strength training alone, exercise therapy alone, and exercise therapy with passive manual mobilisation each reduce pain and disability in people with knee osteoarthritis: a systematic review. *J Physiother* 57, 11-20.

Jensen M., Patterson D.R., 2006. Hypnotic treatment of chronic pain. *J Behav Med* 29, 95-124.

Ji L.L., Gomez-Cabrera M.C., Vina J., 2006. Exercise and hormesis: activation of cellular antioxidant signaling pathway. *Ann N Y Acad Sci* 1067, 425-435.

Jin X.L., Shibata C., Naito H., Ueno T., Funayama Y., Fukushima K., Matsuno S., Sasaki I., 2001. Intraduodenal and intrajejunal administration of the herbal medicine, dai-kenchu-tou, stimulates small intestinal motility via cholinergic receptors in conscious dogs. *Dig Dis Sci* 46, 1171-1176.

Johansen P.O., Krebs T.S., 2009. How could MDMA (ecstasy) help anxiety disorders? A neurobiological rationale. *J Psychopharmacol* 23, 389-391.

John P.J., Sharma N., Sharma C.M., Kankane A., 2007. Effectiveness of yoga therapy in the treatment of migraine without aura: a randomized controlled trial. *Headache* 47, 654-661.

Jong M.C., Jong M.U., Baars E.W., 2012. Adverse drug reactions to anthroposophic and homeopathic solutions for injection: a systematic evaluation of German pharmacovigilance databases. *Pharmacoepidemiol Drug Saf.*

Kabat-Zinn J., Lipworth L., Burney R., 1985. The clinical use of mindfulness meditation for the self-regulation of chronic pain. *J Behav Med* 8, 163-190.

Kamei T., Toriumi Y., Kimura H., Ohno S., Kumano H., Kimura K., 2000. Decrease in serum cortisol during yoga exercise is correlated with alpha wave activation. *Percept Mot Skills* 90, 1027-1032.

Kametani H., Sato A., Sato Y., Simpson A., 1979. Neural mechanisms of reflex facilitation and inhibition of gastric motility to stimulation of various skin areas in rats. *J Physiol* (Lond) 294, 407-418.

Kanji N., White A., Ernst E., 2006. Autogenic training to reduce anxiety in nursing students: randomized controlled trial. *J Adv Nurs* 53, 729-735.

Kantzides A., Owens N.C., De Matteo R., Badoer E., 2005. Right atrial stretch activates neurons in autonomic brain regions that project to the rostral ventrolateral medulla in the rat. *Neuroscience* 133, 775-786.

Kaptchuk T.J., Kelley J.M., Conboy L.A., Davis R.B., Kerr C.E., Jacobson E.E., Kirsch I., Schyner R.N., Nam B.H., Nguyen L.T., Park M., Rivers A.L., McManus C., Kokkotou E., Drossman D.A., Goldman P., Lembo A.J., 2008. Components of placebo effect: randomised controlled trial in patients with irritable bowel syndrome. *Bmj* 336, 999-1003.

Kara M., Ozcakar L., Gokcay D., Ozcelik E., Yorubulut M., Guneri S., Kaymak B., Akinci A., Cetin A., 2010. Quantification of the effects of transcutaneous electrical nerve stimulation with functional magnetic resonance imaging: a double-blind randomized placebo-controlled study. *Arch Phys Med Rehabil* 91, 1160-1165.

Kasl S.V., Cobb S., 1970. Blood pressure changes in men undergoing job loss: a preliminary report. Psychosom Med 32, 19-38.

Kasting N.W., 1988. Simultaneous and independent release of vasopressin and oxytocin in the rat. *Can J Physiol Pharmacol* 66, 22-26.

Kelley D.S., 2001. Modulation of human immune and inflammatory responses by dietary fatty acids. *Nutrition* 17, 669-673.

Kemper K.J., Danhauer S.C., 2005. Music as therapy. *South Med J* 98, 282-288.

Kendrick K.M., Keverne E.B., 1992. Control of synthesis and release of oxytocin in the sheep brain. *Ann N Y Acad Sci* 652, 102-121.

Kerr C.E., Wasserman R.H., Moore C.I., 2007. Cortical dynamics as a therapeutic mechanism for touch healing. *J Altern Complement Med* 13, 59-66.

Kessler R.C., Soukup J., Davis R.B., Foster D.F., Wilkey S.A., Van Rompay M.I., Eisenberg D.M., 2001. The use of complementary and alternative therapies to treat anxiety and depression in the United States. *Am J Psychiatry* 158, 289-294.

Keverne E.B., Martensz N.D., Tuite B., 1989. Beta-endorphin concentrations in cerebrospinal fluid of monkeys are influenced by grooming relationships. *Psychoneuroendocrinology* 14, 155-161.

Khalfa S., Bella S.D., Roy M., Peretz I., Lupien S.J., 2003. Effects of relaxing music on salivary cortisol level after psychological stress. *Ann N Y Acad Sci* 999, 374-376.

Khalsa S.B., Shorter S.M., Cope S., Wyshak G., Sklar E., 2009. Yoga ameliorates performance anxiety and mood disturbance in young professional musicians. *Appl Psychophysiol Biofeedback* 34, 279-289.

Khattab K., Khattab A.A., Ortak J., Richardt G., Bonnemeier H., 2007. Iyengar yoga increases cardiac parasympathetic nervous modulation among healthy yoga practitioners. *Evid Based Complement Alternat Med* 4, 511-517.

Kim M.S., Chey W.D., Owyang C., Hasler W.L., 1997. Role of plasma vasopressin as a mediator of nausea and gastric slow wave dysrhythmias in motion sickness. *Am J Physiol* 272, G853-862.

Kirsch I., Deacon B.J., Huedo-Medina T.B., Scoboria A., Moore T.J., Johnson B.T., 2008. Initial severity and antidepressant benefits: a meta-analysis of data submitted to the Food and Drug Administration. *PLoS Med* 5, e45.

Knost B., Flor H., Braun C., Birbaumer N., 1997. Cerebral processing of words and the development of chronic pain. Psychophysiology 34, 474-481.

Koizumi K., Sato A., Terui N., 1980. Role of somatic afferents in autonomic system control of the intestinal motility. *Brain Res* 182, 85-97.

Kolasinski S.L., Garfinkel M., Tsai A.G., Matz W., Van Dyke A., Schumacher H.R., 2005. Iyengar yoga for treating symptoms of osteoarthritis of the knees: a pilot study. *J Altern Complement Med* 11, 689-693.

Koltyn K.F., 2000. Analgesia following exercise: a review. *Sports Med* 29, 85-98.

Koltyn K.F., 2002. Exercise-induced hypoalgesia and intensity of exercise. *Sports Med* 32, 477-487.

Koltyn K.F., Arbogast R.W., 1998. Perception of pain after resistance exercise. *Br J Sports Med* 32, 20-24.

Koltyn K.F., Umeda M., 2006. Exercise, hypoalgesia and blood pressure. *Sports Med* 36, 207-214.

Komelski M.F., Miyazaki Y., Blieszner R., 2012. Comparing the health status of U.S. taijiquan and qigong practitioners to a national survey sample across ages. *J Altern Complement Med* 18, 281-286.

Kosfeld M., Heinrichs M., Zak P.J., Fischbacher U., Fehr E., 2005. Oxytocin increases trust in humans. *Nature* 435, 673-676.

Kristal A.R., Littman A.J., Benitez D., White E., 2005. Yoga practice is associated with attenuated weight gain in healthy, middle-aged men and women. *Altern Ther Health Med* 11, 28-33.

Krnjevic K., Schwartz S., 1967. The action of gamma-aminobutyric acid on cortical neurones. *Exp Brain Res* 3, 320-336.

Kroenke K., Krebs E.E., Bair M.J., 2009. Pharmacotherapy of chronic pain: a synthesis of recommendations from systematic reviews. *Gen Hosp Psychiatry* 31, 206-219.

Kubota Y., Sato W., Toichi M., Murai T., Okada T., Hayashi A., Sengoku A., 2001. Frontal midline theta rhythm is correlated with cardiac autonomic activities during the performance of an attention demanding meditation procedure. *Brain Res Cogn Brain Res* 11, 281-287.

Kuffler S.W., Edwards C., 1958. Mechanism of gamma aminobutyric acid (GABA) action and its relation to synaptic inhibition. *J Neurophysiol* 21, 589-610.

Kuwahara M., Yayou K., Ishii K., Hashimoto S., Tsubone H., Sugano S., 1994. Power spectral analysis of heart rate variability as a new method for assessing autonomic activity in the rat. *J Electrocardiol* 27, 333-337.

Kwekkeboom K.L., Cherwin C.H., Lee J.W., Wanta B., 2010. Mind-body treatments for the pain-fatigue-sleep disturbance symptom cluster in persons with cancer. *J Pain Symptom Manage* 39, 126-138.

Landgraf R., Hacker R., Buhl H., 1982. Plasma vasopressin and oxytocin in response to exercise and during a day-night cycle in man. *Endokrinologie* 79, 281-291.

Lannersten L., Kosek E., 2010. Dysfunction of endogenous pain inhibition during exercise with painful muscles in patients with shoulder myalgia and fibromyalgia. *Pain* 151, 77-86.

Laskey W., Polosa C., 1988. Characteristics of the sympathetic preganglionic neuron and its synaptic input. *Prog Neurobiol* 31, 47-84.

Lavrencic A., Salobir B.G., Keber I., 2000. Physical training improves flow-mediated dilation in patients with the polymetabolic syndrome. *Arterioscler Thromb Vasc Biol* 20, 551-555.

Lazar S.W., Bush G., Gollub R.L., Fricchione G.L., Khalsa G., Benson H., 2000. Functional brain mapping of the relaxation response and meditation. *Neuroreport* 11, 1581-1585.

Le Bars P.L., Katz M.M., Berman N., Itil T.M., Freedman A.M., Schatzberg A.F., 1997. A placebo-controlled, double-blind, randomized trial of an extract of Ginkgo biloba for dementia. North American EGb Study Group. *Jama* 278, 1327-1332.

Leak J.A., 1999. Herbal Medicine: Is it an Alternative or an Unknown? A Brief Review of Popular Herbals Used by Patients in a Pain and Symptom Management Practice Setting. *Curr Rev Pain* 3, 226-236.

Leardi S., Pietroletti R., Angeloni G., Necozione S., Ranalletta G., Del Gusto B., 2007. Randomized clinical trial examining the effect of music therapy in stress response to day surgery. *Br J Surg* 94, 943-947.

Lee C.H., Jung H.S., Lee T.Y., Lee S.R., Yuk S.W., Lee K.G., Lee B.H., 2001a. Studies of the central neural pathways to the stomach and Zusanli (ST36). *Am J Chin Med* 29, 211-220.

Lee F.H., Raja S.N., 2011. Complementary and alternative medicine in chronic pain. Pain 152, 28-30.

Lee M.S., Pittler M.H., Ernst E., 2007. Is Tai Chi an effective adjunct in cancer care? A systematic review of controlled clinical trials. *Support Care Cancer* 15, 597-601.

Lee M.S., Rim Y.H., Kang C.W., 2004. Effects of external qi-therapy on emotions, electroencephalograms, and plasma cortisol. *Int J Neurosci* 114, 1493-1502.

Lee R.E., Goldberg J.H., Sallis J.F., Hickmann S.A., Castro C.M., Chen A.H., 2001b. A prospective analysis of the relationship between walking and mood in sedentary ethnic minority women. *Women Health* 32, 1-15.

Lehman A.V., 1913. Studien uber reflektorische Darmbewegungen beim Hunde. *Pflugers Arch. Ges. Physiol* 149, 413-433.

Lerman A., Zeiher A.M., 2005. Endothelial function: cardiac events. *Circulation* 111, 363-368.

Leuchter A.F., Cook I.A., Witte E.A., Morgan M., Abrams M., 2002. Changes in brain function of depressed subjects during treatment with placebo. *Am J Psychiatry* 159, 122-129.

Levit K., Smith C., Cowan C., Sensenig A., Catlin A., 2004. Health spending rebound continues in 2002. *Health Aff* 23, 147-159.

Li F., Fisher K.J., Harmer P., Irbe D., Tearse R.G., Weimer C., 2004. Tai chi and self-rated quality of sleep and daytime sleepiness in older adults: a randomized controlled trial. *J Am Geriatr Soc* 52, 892-900.

Li L., Yin-Xiang C., Hong X., Peng L., Da-Nian Z., 2001. Nitric oxide in vPAG mediates the depressor response to acupuncture in stress-induced hypertensive rats. *Acupunct Electrother Res* 26, 165-170.

Li P., Tjen A.L.S.C., Guo Z.L., Fu L.W., Longhurst J.C., 2009. Long-loop pathways in cardiovascular electroacupuncture responses. *J Appl Physiol* 106, 620-630.

Li Y.Q., Zhu B., Rong P.J., Ben H., Li Y.H., 2007. Neural mechanism of acupuncture-modulated gastric motility. *World J Gastroenterol* 13, 709-716.

Libby D.J., Reddy F., Pilver C.E., Desai R.A., 2012. The Use of Yoga in Specialized VA PTSD Treatment Programs. *Int J Yoga Therap,* 79-88.

Lieberman M.D., Jarcho J.M., Berman S., Naliboff B.D., Suyenobu B.Y., Mandelkern M., Mayer E.A., 2004. The neural correlates of placebo effects: a disruption account. *Neuroimage* 22, 447-455.

Lien H.C., Sun W.M., Chen Y.H., Kim H., Hasler W., Owyang C., 2003. Effects of ginger on motion sickness and gastric slow-wave dysrhythmias induced by circular vection. *Am J Physiol Gastrointest Liver Physiol* 284, G481-489.

Light K.C., Grewen K.M., Amico J.A., 2005. More frequent partner hugs and higher oxytocin levels are linked to lower blood pressure and heart rate in premenopausal women. *Biol Psychol* 69, 5-21.

Lin X., Mellow M.H., Southmayd L., 3rd, Pan J., Chen J.D., 1997. Impaired gastric myoelectrical activity in patients with chronic renal failure. *Dig Dis Sci* 42, 898-906.

Linde K., Witt C.M., Streng A., Weidenhammer W., Wagenpfeil S., Brinkhaus B., Willich S.N., Melchart D., 2007. The impact of patient expectations on outcomes in four randomized controlled trials of acupuncture in patients with chronic pain. *Pain* 128, 264-271.

Little S.A., Kligler B., Homel P., Belisle S.S., Merrell W., 2009. Multimodal mind/body group therapy for chronic depression: a pilot study. *Explore* (NY) 5, 330-337.

Liu J.H., Li J., Yan J., Chang X.R., Cui R.F., He J.F., Hu J.M., 2004a. Expression of c-fos in the nucleus of the solitary tract following electroacupuncture at facial acupoints and gastric distension in rats. *Neurosci Lett* 366, 215-219.

Liu S., Peng S., Hou X., Ke M., Chen J.D., 2008. Transcutaneous electroacupuncture improves dyspeptic symptoms and increases high frequency heart rate variability in patients with functional dyspepsia. *Neurogastroenterol Motil* 20, 1204-1211.

Liu W.C., Feldman S.C., Cook D.B., Hung D.L., Xu T., Kalnin A.J., Komisaruk B.R., 2004b. fMRI study of acupuncture-induced periaqueductal gray activity in humans. Neuroreport 15, 1937-1940.

Liu Y., Mimura K., Wang L., Ikuta K., 2005. Psychological and physiological effects of 24-style taijiquan. *Neuropsychobiology* 52, 212-218.

Louvel D., Delvaux M., Felez A., Fioramonti J., Bueno L., Lazorthes Y., Frexinos J., 1996. Oxytocin increases thresholds of colonic visceral perception in patients with irritable bowel syndrome. *Gut* 39, 741-747.

Lu B., Chow A., 1999. Neurotrophins and hippocampal synaptic transmission and plasticity. *J Neurosci Res* 58, 76-87.

Lu W.A., Kuo C.D., 2003. The effect of Tai Chi Chuan on the autonomic nervous modulation in older persons. *Med Sci Sports Exerc* 35, 1972-1976.

Lund I., Ge Y., Yu L.C., Uvnas-Moberg K., Wang J., Yu C., Kurosawa M., Agren G., Rosen A., Lekman M., Lundeberg T., 2002. Repeated massage-like stimulation induces long-term effects on nociception: contribution of oxytocinergic mechanisms. *Eur J Neurosci* 16, 330-338.

Lutz A., Slagter H.A., Dunne J.D., Davidson R.J., 2008. Attention regulation and monitoring in meditation. *Trends Cogn Sci* 12, 163-169.

Ma X.P., Tan L.Y., Yang Y., Wu H.G., Jiang B., Liu H.R., Yang L., 2009. Effect of electro-acupuncture on substance P, its receptor and corticotropin-releasing hormone in rats with irritable bowel syndrome. *World J Gastroenterol* 15, 5211-5217.

MacMahon S., Kermode S., 1998. A clinical trial of the effect of aromatherapy on motivational behaviour in a dementia care setting using a single subject design. *Aust J Holist Nurs* 5, 47-49.

Madanmohan, Udupa K., Bhavanani A.B., Shatapathy C.C., Sahai A., 2004. Modulation of cardiovascular response to exercise by yoga training. *Indian J Physiol Pharmacol* 48, 461-465.

Maiorana A., O'Driscoll G., Cheetham C., Dembo L., Stanton K., Goodman C., Taylor R., Green D., 2001. The effect of combined aerobic and resistance exercise training on vascular function in type 2 diabetes. *J Am Coll Cardiol* 38, 860-866.

Malkin K., 1994. Use of massage in clinical practice. Br J Nurs 3, 292-294.

Manabe N., Camilleri M., Rao A., Wong B.S., Burton D., Busciglio I., Zinsmeister A.R., Haruma K., 2010. Effect of daikenchuto (TU-100) on gastrointestinal and colonic transit in humans. *Am J Physiol Gastrointest Liver Physiol* 298, G970-975.

Manchanda S.C., Narang R., Reddy K.S., Sachdeva U., Prabhakaran D., Dharmanand S., Rajani M., Bijlani R., 2000. Retardation of coronary atherosclerosis with yoga lifestyle intervention. *J Assoc Physicians India* 48, 687-694.

Manheimer E., Linde K., Lao L., Bouter L.M., Berman B.M., 2007. Meta-analysis: acupuncture for osteoarthritis of the knee. *Ann Intern Med* 146, 868-877.

Manjunath N.K., Telles S., 2005. Influence of Yoga and Ayurveda on self-rated sleep in a geriatric population. Indian J Med Res 121, 683-690.

Manni L., Aloe L., Fiore M., 2009. Changes in cognition induced by social isolation in the mouse are restored by electro-acupuncture. Physiol Behav 98, 537-542.

Marchand W.R., 2012. Mindfulness-based stress reduction, mindfulness-based cognitive therapy, and Zen meditation for depression, anxiety, pain, and psychological distress. J Psychiatr Pract 18, 233-252.

Marmot M.G., Syme S.L., Kagan A., Kato H., Cohen J.B., Belsky J., 1975. Epidemiologic studies of coronary heart disease and stroke in Japanese men living in Japan, Hawaii and California: prevalence of coronary and hypertensive heart disease and associated risk factors. *Am J Epidemiol* 102, 514-525.

Martin B.I., Deyo R.A., Mirza S.K., Turner J.A., Comstock B.A., Hollingworth W., Sullivan S.D., 2008. Expenditures and health status among adults with back and neck problems. *Jama* 299, 656-664.

Matthiesen A.S., Ransjo-Arvidson A.B., Nissen E., Uvnas-Moberg K., 2001. Postpartum maternal oxytocin release by newborns: effects of infant hand massage and sucking. *Birth* 28, 13-19.

Mayberg H.S., Silva J.A., Brannan S.K., Tekell J.L., Mahurin R.K., McGinnis S., Jerabek P.A., 2002. The functional neuroanatomy of the placebo effect. *Am J Psychiatry* 159, 728-737.

McAuley E., Blissmer B., 2000a. Self-efficacy determinants and consequences of physical activity. *Exerc Sport Sci Rev* 28, 85-88.

McAuley E., Blissmer B., Katula J., Duncan T.E., Mihalko S.L., 2000b. Physical activity, self-esteem, and self-efficacy relationships in older adults: a randomized controlled trial. *Ann Behav Med* 22, 131-139.

McFadden K.L., Hernandez T.D., 2010. Cardiovascular benefits of acupressure (Jin Shin) following stroke. *Complement Ther Med* 18, 42-48.

McGlone F., Vallbo A.B., Olausson H., Loken L., Wessberg J., 2007. Discriminative touch and emotional touch. *Can J Exp Psychol* 61, 173-183.

McIver S., McGartland M., O'Halloran P., 2009. "Overeating is not about the food": women describe their experience of a yoga treatment program for binge eating. *Qual Health Res* 19, 1234-1245.

Medalie J.H., Goldbourt U., 1976. Angina pectoris among 10,000 men. II. Psychosocial and other risk factors as evidenced by a multivariate analysis of a five year incidence study. *Am J Med* 60, 910-921.

Medical-Malprocess, 2010. Capitalism in Healthcare–Yes or No? http://thesystemmd.com/?p=1200.

Meeker W.C., Haldeman S., 2002. Chiropractic: a profession at the crossroads of mainstream and alternative medicine. *Ann Intern Med* 136, 216-227.

Meeus M., Roussel N.A., Truijen S., Nijs J., 2010. Reduced pressure pain thresholds in response to exercise in chronic fatigue syndrome but not in chronic low back pain: an experimental study. *J Rehabil Med* 42, 884-890.

Melzack R., Stillwell D.M., Fox E.J., 1977. Trigger points and acupuncture points for pain: correlations and implications. *Pain* 3, 3-23.

Melzack R., Wall P.D., 1965. Pain mechanisms: a new theory. *Science* 150, 971-979.

Menetrey D., Basbaum A.I., 1987. Spinal and trigeminal projections to the nucleus of the solitary tract: a possible substrate for somatovisceral and viscerovisceral reflex activation. J Comp Neurol 255, 439-450.

Meston C.M., Frohlich P.F., 2000. The neurobiology of sexual function. *Arch Gen Psychiatry* 57, 1012-1030.

Michalsen A., Grossman P., Acil A., Langhorst J., Ludtke R., Esch T., Stefano G.B., Dobos G.J., 2005. Rapid stress reduction and anxiolysis among distressed women as a consequence of a three-month intensive yoga program. *Med Sci Monit* 11, CR555-561.

Michelini L.C., 2001. Oxytocin in the NTS. A new modulator of cardiovascular control during exercise. *Ann N Y Acad* Sci 940, 206-220.

Millan M.J., 2002. Descending control of pain. Prog Neurobiol 66, 355-474.

Miller L.A., 2009. Oxytocin, excessive uterine activity, and patient safety: time for a collaborative approach. *J Perinat Neonatal Nurs* 23, 52-58.

Miluk-Kolasa B., Obminski Z., Stupnicki R., Golec L., 1994. Effects of music treatment on salivary cortisol in patients exposed to pre-surgical stress. *Exp Clin Endocrinol* 102, 118-120.

Missig G., Ayers L.W., Schulkin J., Rosen J.B., 2010. Oxytocin reduces background anxiety in a fear-potentiated startle paradigm. *Neuropsychopharmacology* 35, 2607-2616.

Mitsui S., Yamamoto M., Nagasawa M., Mogi K., Kikusui T., Ohtani N., Ohta M., 2011. Urinary oxytocin as a noninvasive biomarker of positive emotion in dogs. *Horm Behav* 60, 239-243.

Mittleman M.A., Maclure M., Sherwood J.B., Mulry R.P., Tofler G.H., Jacobs S.C., Friedman R., Benson H., Muller J.E., 1995. Triggering of acute myocardial infarction onset by episodes of anger. Determinants of Myocardial Infarction Onset Study Investigators. *Circulation* 92, 1720-1725.

Mohri Y., Fumoto M., Sato-Suzuki I., Umino M., Arita H., 2005. Prolonged rhythmic gum chewing suppresses nociceptive response via serotonergic descending inhibitory pathway in humans. *Pain* 118, 35-42.

Mok E., Wong K.Y., 2003. Effects of music on patient anxiety. *AORN* J 77, 396-397, 401-396, 409-310.

Mommaerts J.L., Devroey D., 2012. The placebo effect: how the subconscious fits in. *Perspect Biol Med* 55, 43-58.

Montgomery G.H., Hallquist M.N., Schnur J.B., David D., Silverstein J.H., Bovbjerg D.H., 2010. Mediators of a brief hypnosis intervention to control side effects in breast surgery patients: response expectancies and emotional distress. *J Consult Clin Psychol* 78, 80-88.

Morhenna V., Park J., Piper E., Zakb P., 2008 Monetary sacrifice among strangers is mediated by endogenous oxytocin release after physical contact. *Evol Hum Behav* 29, 375–383.

Morone N.E., Greco C.M., Weiner D.K., 2008. Mindfulness meditation for the treatment of chronic low back pain in older adults: a randomized controlled pilot study. *Pain* 134, 310-319.

Motivala S.J., Sollers J., Thayer J., Irwin M.R., 2006. Tai Chi Chih acutely decreases sympathetic nervous system activity in older adults. *J Gerontol A Biol Sci Med Sci* 61, 1177-1180.

Moyer C.A., Rounds J., Hannum J.W., 2004. A meta-analysis of massage therapy research. *Psychol Bull* 130, 3-18.

Mueller D.P., 1980. Social networks: a promising direction for research on the relationship of the social environment to psychiatric disorder. *Soc Sci Med Med Psychol Med Sociol* 14A, 147-161.

Mukaddam-Daher S., Yin Y.L., Roy J., Gutkowska J., Cardinal R., 2001. Negative inotropic and chronotropic effects of oxytocin. *Hypertension* 38, 292-296.

Mukherjee P.K., Ponnusankar S., Pandit S., Hazam P.K., Ahmmed M., Mukherjee K., 2011. Botanicals as medicinal food and their effects on drug metabolizing enzymes. *Food Chem Toxicol* 49, 3142-3153.

Mustian K.M., Katula J.A., Zhao H., 2006. A pilot study to assess the influence of tai chi chuan on functional capacity among breast cancer survivors. *J Support Oncol* 4, 139-145.

Mustian K.M., Palesh O.G., Flecksteiner S.A., 2008. Tai Chi Chuan for breast cancer survivors. *Med Sport Sci* 52, 209-217.

Nabkasorn C., Miyai N., Sootmongkol A., Junprasert S., Yamamoto H., Arita M., Miyashita K., 2006. Effects of physical exercise on depression, neuroendocrine stress hormones and physiological fitness in adolescent females with depressive symptoms. *Eur J Public Health* 16, 179-184.

Napadow V., Dhond R.P., Kim J., LaCount L., Vangel M., Harris R.E., Kettner N., Park K., 2009. Brain encoding of acupuncture sensation--coupling on-line rating with fMRI. *Neuroimage* 47, 1055-1065.

Neumann I.D., 2008. Brain oxytocin: a key regulator of emotional and social behaviours in both females and males. *J Neuroendocrinol* 20, 858-865.

Nijs J., Kosek E., Van Oosterwijck J., Meeus M., 2012. Dysfunctional endogenous analgesia during exercise in patients with chronic pain: to exercise or not to exercise? *Pain Physician* 15, ES205-213.

Nilsson U., 2009. Soothing music can increase oxytocin levels during bed rest after open-heart surgery: a randomised control trial. *J Clin Nurs* 18, 2153-2161.

Nilsson U., Rawal N., Unosson M., 2003. A comparison of intra-operative or postoperative exposure to music--a controlled trial of the effects on postoperative pain. *Anaesthesia* 58, 699-703.

Nilsson U., Unosson M., Rawal N., 2005. Stress reduction and analgesia in patients exposed to calming music postoperatively: a randomized controlled trial. *Eur J Anaesthesiol* 22, 96-102.

Nordmann J.J., Dayanithi G., 1988. Release of neuropeptides does not only occur at nerve terminals. *Biosci Rep* 8, 471-483.

Norman G.J., Karelina K., Morris J.S., Zhang N., Cochran M., Courtney DeVries A., 2010. Social interaction prevents the development of depressive-like behavior post nerve injury in mice: a potential role for oxytocin. *Psychosom Med* 72, 519-526.

Ohayon M.M., Shapiro C.M., 2000. Sleep disturbances and psychiatric disorders associated with posttraumatic stress disorder in the general population. Compr Psychiatry 41, 469-478.

Okamoto Y., Ohtani N., Uchiyama H., Ohta M., 2009. The feeding behavior of dogs correlates with their responses to commands. *J Vet Med Sci* 71, 1617-1621.

Oken B.S., Zajdel D., Kishiyama S., Flegal K., Dehen C., Haas M., Kraemer D.F., Lawrence J., Leyva J., 2006. Randomized, controlled, six-month trial of yoga in healthy seniors: effects on cognition and quality of life. *Altern Ther Health Med* 12, 40-47.

Olausson H., Lamarre Y., Backlund H., Morin C., Wallin B.G., Starck G., Ekholm S., Strigo I., Worsley K., Vallbo A.B., Bushnell M.C., 2002. Unmyelinated tactile afferents signal touch and project to insular cortex. *Nat Neurosci* 5, 900-904.

Olff M., Langeland W., Witteveen A., Denys D., 2010. A psychobiological rationale for oxytocin in the treatment of posttraumatic stress disorder. *CNS Spectr* 15, 522-530.

Ondrejcakova M., Ravingerova T., Bakos J., Pancza D., Jezova D., 2009. Oxytocin exerts protective effects on in vitro myocardial injury induced by ischemia and reperfusion. *Can J Physiol Pharmacol* 87, 137-142.

Ospina M.B., Bond K., Karkhaneh M., Buscemi N., Dryden D.M., Barnes V., Carlson L.E., Dusek J.A., Shannahoff-Khalsa D., 2008. Clinical trials of meditation practices in health care: characteristics and quality. *J Altern Complement Med* 14, 1199-1213.

Ospina M.B., Bond K., Karkhaneh M., Tjosvold L., Vandermeer B., Liang Y., Bialy L., Hooton N., Buscemi N., Dryden D.M., Klassen T.P., 2007. Meditation practices for health: state of the research. *Evid Rep Technol Assess* (Full Rep), 1-263.

Panagiotakos D.B., Chrysohoou C., Siasos G., Zisimos K., Skoumas J., Pitsavos C., Stefanadis C., 2011. Sociodemographic and lifestyle statistics of oldest old people (>80 years) living in ikaria island: the ikaria study. *Cardiol Res Pract* 2011, 679187.

Panjabi M.M., 2006. A hypothesis of chronic back pain: ligament subfailure injuries lead to muscle control dysfunction. *Eur Spine J* 15, 668-676.

Pariente J., White P., Frackowiak R.S., Lewith G., 2005. Expectancy and belief modulate the neuronal substrates of pain treated by acupuncture. *Neuroimage* 25, 1161-1167.

Patel S.M., Stason W.B., Legedza A., Ock S.M., Kaptchuk T.J., Conboy L., Canenguez K., Park J.K., Kelly E., Jacobson E., Kerr C.E., Lembo A.J., 2005. The placebo effect in irritable bowel syndrome trials: a meta-analysis. *Neurogastroenterol Motil* 17, 332-340.

Patra S., Telles S., 2010. Heart rate variability during sleep following the practice of cyclic meditation and supine rest. *Appl Psychophysiol Biofeedback* 35, 135-140.

Pattison N., Warren L., 2003. 2002 drug industry profits: hefty pharmaceutical company margins dwarf other industries. Washington (DC): Public Citizen Congress Watch; June. www.citizen.org/documents/ Pharma_Report.pdf.

Paul-Labrador M., Polk D., Dwyer J.H., Velasquez I., Nidich S., Rainforth M., Schneider R., Merz C.N., 2006. Effects of a randomized controlled trial of transcendental meditation on components of the metabolic syndrome in subjects with coronary heart disease. *Arch Intern Med* 166, 1218-1224.

Peppone L.J., Mustian K.M., Janelsins M.C., Palesh O.G., Rosier R.N., Piazza K.M., Purnell J.Q., Darling T.V., Morrow G.R., 2010. Effects of a structured weight-bearing exercise program on bone metabolism among breast cancer survivors: a feasibility trial. *Clin Breast Cancer* 10, 224-229.

Petersson M., 2002. Cardiovascular effects of oxytocin. *Prog Brain Res* 139, 281-288.

Petersson M., Lundeberg T., Uvnas-Moberg K., 1999. Short-term increase and long-term decrease of blood pressure in response to oxytocin-potentiating effect of female steroid hormones. *J Cardiovasc Pharmacol* 33, 102-108.

Petrovic P., Kalso E., Petersson K.M., Andersson J., Fransson P., Ingvar M., 2011. A prefrontal non-opioid mechanism in placebo analgesia. *Pain* 150, 59-65.

Petrovic P., Kalso E., Petersson K.M., Ingvar M., 2002. Placebo and opioid analgesia-- imaging a shared neuronal network. *Science* 295, 1737-1740.

Phan K.L., Fitzgerald D.A., Nathan P.J., Tancer M.E., 2006. Association between amygdala hyperactivity to harsh faces and severity of social anxiety in generalized social phobia. *Biol Psychiatry* 59, 424-429.

Phongsuphap S., Pongsupap Y., Chandanamattha P., Lursinsap C., 2008. Changes in heart rate variability during concentration meditation. *Int J Cardiol* 130, 481-484.

Pickar J.G., Bolton P.S., 2012. Spinal manipulative therapy and somatosensory activation. *J Electromyogr Kinesiol* 22, 785-794.

Piliavin J.A., Siegl E., 2007. Health benefits of volunteering in the Wisconsin longitudinal study. *J Health Soc Behav* 48, 450-464.

Pilkington K., 2010. Anxiety, depression and acupuncture: A review of the clinical research. *Auton Neurosci* 157, 91-95.

Pomeranz B., Macaulay R.J., Caudill M.A., Kutz I., Adam D., Gordon D., Kilborn K.M., Barger A.C., Shannon D.C., Cohen R.J., Benson H., 1985. Assessment of autonomic function in humans by heart rate spectral analysis. *Am J Physiol* 248, H151-153.

Porzio G., Trapasso T., Martelli S., Sallusti E., Piccone C., Mattei A., Di Stanislao C., Ficorella C., Marchetti P., 2002. Acupuncture in the treatment of menopause-related symptoms in women taking tamoxifen. *Tumori* 88, 128-130.

Posner M.I., Rothbart M.K., Sheese B.E., Tang Y., 2007. The anterior cingulate gyrus and the mechanism of self-regulation. *Cogn Affect Behav Neurosci* 7, 391-395.

Potts J.T., 2001. Exercise and sensory integration. Role of the nucleus tractus solitarius. *Ann N Y Acad Sci* 940, 221-236.

Potts J.T., Paton J.F., Mitchell J.H., Garry M.G., Kline G., Anguelov P.T., Lee S.M., 2003. Contraction-sensitive skeletal muscle afferents inhibit arterial baroreceptor signalling in the nucleus of the solitary tract: role of intrinsic GABA interneurons. *Neuroscience* 119, 201-214.

Price D.D., Craggs J., Verne G.N., Perlstein W.M., Robinson M.E., 2007. Placebo analgesia is accompanied by large reductions in pain-related brain activity in irritable bowel syndrome patients. Pain 127, 63-72.

Priest P., 2007. The healing balm effect: using a walking group to feel better. *J Health Psychol* 12, 36-52.

Prior A., Colgan S., Whorwell P., 1990a. Changes in rectal sensitivity after hypnotherapy in patients with irritable bowel syndrome. *Gut* 31, 896-898.

Prior A., Colgan S.M., Whorwell P.J., 1990b. Changes in rectal sensitivity after hypnotherapy in patients with irritable bowel syndrome. Gut 31, 896-898.

Radak Z., Chung H.Y., Goto S., 2005. Exercise and hormesis: oxidative stress-related adaptation for successful aging. *Biogerontology* 6, 71-75.

Ransford C.P., 1982. A role for amines in the antidepressant effect of exercise: a review. *Med Sci Sports Exerc* 14, 1-10.

Rao M.R., Raghuram N., Nagendra H.R., Gopinath K.S., Srinath B.S., Diwakar R.B., Patil S., Bilimagga S.R., Rao N., Varambally S., 2009. Anxiolytic effects of a yoga program in early breast cancer patients undergoing conventional treatment: a randomized controlled trial. *Complement Ther Med* 17, 1-8.

Rapaport M.H., Schettler P., Bresee C., 2012. A preliminary study of the effects of repeated massage on hypothalamic-pituitary-adrenal and immune function in healthy individuals: a study of mechanisms of action and dosage. *J Altern Complement Med* 18, 789-797.

Ray C.A., Carter J.R., 2007. Central modulation of exercise-induced muscle pain in humans. *J Physiol* 585, 287-294.

Relman A., 2001. Separating continuing medical education from pharmaceutical marketing. *JAMA* 285, 2009-2012.

Rennie K.L., Hughes J., Lang R., Jebb S.A., 2003. Nutritional management of rheumatoid arthritis: a review of the evidence. *J Hum Nutr Diet* 16, 97-109.

Renzi C., Peticca L., Pescatori M., 2000. The use of relaxation techniques in the perioperative management of proctological patients: preliminary results. *Int J Colorectal Di*s 15, 313-316.

Ring R.H., Malberg J.E., Potestio L., Ping J., Boikess S., Luo B., Schechter L.E., Rizzo S., Rahman Z., Rosenzweig-Lipson S., 2006. Anxiolytic-like activity of oxytocin in male mice: behavioral and autonomic evidence, therapeutic implications. *Psychopharmacology* (Berl) 185, 218-225.

Roelofs P.D., Deyo R.A., Koes B.W., Scholten R.J., van Tulder M.W., 2008. Non-steroidal anti-inflammatory drugs for low back pain. *Cochrane Database Syst Rev,* CD000396.

Rojas-Piloni G., Mejia-Rodriguez R., Martinez-Lorenzana G., Condes-Lara M., 2010. Oxytocin, but not vassopressin, modulates nociceptive responses in dorsal horn neurons. *Neurosci Lett* 476, 32-35.

Roland B.L., Sawchenko P.E., 1993. Local origins of some GABAergic projections to the paraventricular and supraoptic nuclei of the hypothalamus in the rat. *J Comp Neurol* 332, 123-143.

Rosenberg E.I., Genao I., Chen I., Mechaber A.J., Wood J.A., Faselis C.J., Kurz J., Menon M., O'Rorke J., Panda M., Pasanen M., Staton L., Calleson D., Cykert S., 2008. Complementary and alternative medicine use by primary care patients with chronic pain. *Pain Med* 9, 1065-1072.

Rowe J.W., Shelton R.L., Helderman J.H., Vestal R.E., Robertson G.L., 1979. Influence of the emetic reflex on vasopressin release in man. *Kidney Int* 16, 729-735.

Ruberman W., Weinblatt E., Goldberg J.D., Chaudhary B.S., 1984. Psychosocial influences on mortality after myocardial infarction. *N Engl J Med* 311, 552-559.

Ruis M.A., te Brake J.H., Buwalda B., De Boer S.F., Meerlo P., Korte S.M., Blokhuis H.J., Koolhaas J.M., 1999. Housing familiar male wildtype rats together reduces the long-term adverse behavioural and physiological effects of social defeat. *Psychoneuroendocrinology* 24, 285-300.

Ruscio M.G., Sweeny T., Hazelton J., Suppatkul P., Sue Carter C., 2007. Social environment regulates corticotropin releasing factor, corticosterone and vasopressin in juvenile prairie voles. *Horm Behav* 51, 54-61.

Sallam H., McNearney T.A., Doshi D., Chen J.D., 2007. Transcutaneous electrical nerve stimulation (TENS) improves upper GI symptoms and balances the sympathovagal activity in scleroderma patients. *Dig Dis Sci* 52, 1329-1337.

Salonia A., Nappi R.E., Pontillo M., Daverio R., Smeraldi A., Briganti A., Fabbri F., Zanni G., Rigatti P., Montorsi F., 2005. Menstrual cycle-related changes in plasma oxytocin are relevant to normal sexual function in healthy women. *Horm Behav* 47, 164-169.

Salzberg S., 1995. Loving-kindness. Shambala, Boston, MA.

Sansone G.R., Gerdes C.A., Steinman J.L., Winslow J.T., Ottenweller J.E., Komisaruk B.R., Insel T.R., 2002. Vaginocervical stimulation releases oxytocin within the spinal cord in rats. *Neuroendocrinology* 75, 306-315.

Saper R.B., Sherman K.J., Cullum-Dugan D., Davis R.B., Phillips R.S., Culpepper L., 2009. Yoga for chronic low back pain in a predominantly minority population: a pilot randomized controlled trial. *Altern Ther Health Med* 15, 18-27.

Saps M., Youssef N., Miranda A., Nurko S., Hyman P., Cocjin J., Di Lorenzo C., 2009. Multicenter, randomized, placebo-controlled trial of amitriptyline in children with functional gastrointestinal disorders. *Gastroenterology* 137, 1261-1269.

Sarang P.S., Telles S., 2006. Oxygen consumption and respiration during and after two yoga relaxation techniques. *Appl Psychophysiol Biofeedback* 31, 143-153.

Sato A., Sato Y., Shimada F., Torigata Y., 1975. Changes in gastric motility produced by nociceptive stimulation of the skin rats. *Brain Res* 87, 151-159.

Sato A., Sato Y., Suzuki A., Uchida S., 1993. Neural mechanisms of the reflex inhibition and excitation of gastric motility elicited by acupuncture-like stimulation in anesthetized rats. *Neurosci Res* 18, 53-62.

Sauro M.D., Greenberg R.P., 2005. Endogenous opiates and the placebo effect: a meta-analytic review. *J Psychosom Res* 58, 115-120.

Schachner L., Field T., Hernandez-Reif M., Duarte A.M., Krasnegor J., 1998. Atopic dermatitis symptoms decreased in children following massage therapy. *Pediatr Dermatol* 15, 390-395.

Schlamann M., Naglatzki R., de Greiff A., Forsting M., Gizewski E.R., 2010. Autogenic training alters cerebral activation patterns in fMRI. *Int J Clin Exp Hypn* 58, 444-456.

Schmid A.A., Van Puymbroeck M., Koceja D.M., 2010. Effect of a 12-week yoga intervention on fear of falling and balance in older adults: a pilot study. *Arch Phys Med Rehabil* 91, 576-583.

Schneider R.H., Alexander C.N., Staggers F., Rainforth M., Salerno J.W., Hartz A., Arndt S., Barnes V.A., Nidich S.I., 2005. Long-term effects of stress reduction on mortality in persons > or = 55 years of age with systemic hypertension. *Am J Cardiol* 95, 1060-1064.

Schneiderman I., Zagoory-Sharon O., Leckman J.F., Feldman R., 2012. Oxytocin during the initial stages of romantic attachment: Relations to couples' interactive reciprocity. *Psychoneuroendocrinology*.

Seeman T.E., 1996. Social ties and health: the benefits of social integration. Ann Epidemiol 6, 442-451.

Segal Z.V., Pearson J.L., Thase M.E., 2003. Challenges in preventing relapse in major depression. Report of a National Institute of Mental Health Workshop on state of the science of relapse prevention in major depression. *J Affect Disord* 77, 97-108.

Seltzer L.J., Ziegler T.E., Pollak S.D., 2010. Social vocalizations can release oxytocin in humans. Proc Biol Sci 277, 2661-2666.

Selvamurthy W., Sridharan K., Ray U.S., Tiwary R.S., Hegde K.S., Radhakrishan U., Sinha K.C., 1998. A new physiological approach to control essential hypertension. *Indian J Physiol Pharmacol* 42, 205-213.

Shapiro D., Cook I.A., Davydov D.M., Ottaviani C., Leuchter A.F., Abrams M., 2007. Yoga as a complementary treatment of depression: effects of traits and moods on treatment outcome. *Evid Based Complement Alternat Med* 4, 493-502.

Shapiro S.L., Carlson L.E., Astin J.A., Freedman B., 2006. Mechanisms of mindfulness. *J Clin Psychol* 62, 373-386.

Sharp J.L., Zammit T.G., Azar T.A., Lawson D.M., 2002. Stress-like responses to common procedures in male rats housed alone or with other rats. *Contemp Top Lab Anim Sci* 41, 8-14.

Sheehan P.W., 1980. Factors influencing rapport in hypnosis. *J Abnorm Psychol* 89, 563-581.

Shelov D.V., Suchday S., Friedberg J.P., 2009. A pilot study measuring the impact of yoga on the trait of mindfulness. *Behav Cogn Psychother* 37, 595-598.

Sher L., 1998. The endogenous euphoric reward system that reinforces physical training: a mechanism for mankind's survival. *Med Hypotheses* 51, 449-450.

Sherman K.J., Cherkin D.C., Erro J., Miglioretti D.L., Deyo R.A., 2005. Comparing yoga, exercise, and a self-care book for chronic low back pain: a randomized, controlled trial. *Ann Intern Med* 143, 849-856.

Silagy C.A., Neil H.A., 1994. A meta-analysis of the effect of garlic on blood pressure. *J Hypertens* 12, 463-468.

Singh D., Gupta R., Saraf S.A., 2011. Herbs-are they safe enough? an overview. *Crit Rev Food Sci Nutr* 52, 876-898.

Singh R.B., Dubnov G., Niaz M.A., Ghosh S., Singh R., Rastogi S.S., Manor O., Pella D., Berry E.M., 2002. Effect of an Indo-Mediterranean diet on progression of coronary artery disease in high risk patients (Indo-Mediterranean Diet Heart Study): a randomised single-blind trial. *Lancet* 360, 1455-1461.

Slater J., Hunt H.T., 1997. Postural-vestibular integration and forms of dreaming: a preliminary report on the effects of brief T'ai Chi Chuan training. *Percept Mot Skills* 85, 97-98.

Sloman R., Brown P., Aldana E., Chee E., 1994. The use of relaxation for the promotion of comfort and pain relief in persons with advanced cancer. *Contemp Nurse* 3, 6-12.

Sluka K.A., Walsh D., 2003. Transcutaneous electrical nerve stimulation: basic science mechanisms and clinical effectiveness. *J Pain* 4, 109-121.

Smith C.A., Hay P.P., Macpherson H., 2010. Acupuncture for depression. *Cochrane Database Syst Rev*, CD004046.

Smith J.C., Joyce C.A., 2004. Mozart versus new age music: relaxation states, stress, and ABC relaxation theory. *J Music Ther* 41, 215-224.

Speed-Andrews A.E., Stevinson C., Belanger L.J., Mirus J.J., Courneya K.S., 2010. Pilot evaluation of an Iyengar yoga program for breast cancer survivors. *Cancer Nurs* 33, 369-381.

Spencer R., Beaumont E., Del Carmen M., Growdon W., Goodman A., 2012. Acupuncture for chemotherapy-induced nausea and vomiting. *Medical Acupuncture* 24, 104-112.

Spiegel D., 1983. Hypnosis with medical/surgical patients. *Gen Hosp Psychiatry* 5, 265-277.

Spiegel D., Giese-Davis J., 2003. Depression and cancer: mechanisms and disease progression. *Biol Psychiatry* 54, 269-282.

Sprod L.K., Janelsins M.C., Palesh O.G., Carroll J.K., Heckler C.E., Peppone L.J., Mohile S.G., Morrow G.R., Mustian K.M., 2012. Health-related quality of life and biomarkers in breast cancer survivors participating in tai chi chuan. *J Cancer Surviv* 6, 146-154.

Srbely J.Z., Dickey J.P., Lee D., Lowerison M., 2010. Dry needle stimulation of myofascial trigger points evokes segmental anti-nociceptive effects. *J Rehabil Med* 42, 463-468.

Stake-Nilsson K., Hultcrantz R., Unge P., Wengstrom Y., 2011. Complementary and alternative medicine used by persons with functional gastrointestinal disorders to alleviate symptom distress. *J Clin Nurs* 21, 800-808.

Stanger M.J., Thompson L.A., Young A.J., Lieberman H.R., 2011. Anticoagulant activity of select dietary supplements. *Nutr Rev* 70, 107-117.

Stein C., Reinecke H., Sorgatz H., 2010. Opioid use in chronic noncancer pain: guidelines revisited. *Curr Opin Anaesthesiol* 23, 598-601.

Stein D.J., Vythilingum B., 2009. Love and attachment: the psychobiology of social bonding. *CNS Spectr* 14, 239-242.

Stephenson N.L., Weinrich S.P., Tavakoli A.S., 2000. The effects of foot reflexology on anxiety and pain in patients with breast and lung cancer. *Oncol Nurs Forum* 27, 67-72.

Stewart J.H., 2005. Hypnosis in contemporary medicine. Mayo Clin Proc 80, 511-524.

Stewart M.J., Maher C.G., Refshauge K.M., Herbert R.D., Bogduk N., Nicholas M., 2007. Randomized controlled trial of exercise for chronic whiplash-associated disorders. *Pain* 128, 59-68.

Stock S., Uvnas-Moberg K., 1988. Increased plasma levels of oxytocin in response to afferent electrical stimulation of the sciatic and vagal nerves and in response to touch and pinch in anaesthetized rats. *Acta Physiol Scand* 132, 29-34.

Strathearn L., Fonagy P., Amico J., Montague P.R., 2009. Adult attachment predicts maternal brain and oxytocin response to infant cues. *Neuropsychopharmacology* 34, 2655-2666.

Street R.L., Jr., Makoul G., Arora N.K., Epstein R.M., 2009. How does communication heal? Pathways linking clinician-patient communication to health outcomes. *Patient Educ Couns* 74, 295-301.

Stux G., Pomeranz B., 1995. Basics of Acupuncture. Fourth edition, Springer NY.

Suarez-Almazor M.E., Looney C., Liu Y., Cox V., Pietz K., Marcus D.M., Street R.L., Jr., 2010. A randomized controlled trial of acupuncture for osteoarthritis of the knee: effects of patient-provider communication. *Arthritis Care Re*s (Hoboken) 62, 1229-1236.

Sun Y., Gan T.J., 2008a. Acupuncture for the management of chronic headache: a systematic review. *Anesth Analg* 107, 2038-2047.

Sun Y., Gan T.J., Dubose J.W., Habib A.S., 2008b. Acupuncture and related techniques for postoperative pain: a systematic review of randomized controlled trials. *Br J Anaesth* 101, 151-160

Suzuki T., Takayama K., Miura M., 1997. Distribution and projection of the medullary cardiovascular control neurons containing glutamate, glutamic acid decarboxylase, tyrosine hydroxylase and phenylethanolamine N-methyltransferase in rats. *Neurosci Res* 27, 9-19.

Sweetser S., Camilleri M., Linker Nord S.J., Burton D.D., Castenada L., Croop R., Tong G., Dockens R., Zinsmeister A.R., 2009. Do corticotropin releasing factor-1 receptors influence colonic transit and bowel function in women with irritable bowel syndrome? *Am J Physiol Gastrointest Liver Physiol* 296, G1299-1306.

Syrjala K.L., Cummings C., Donaldson G.W., 1992. Hypnosis or cognitive behavioral training for the reduction of pain and nausea during cancer treatment: a controlled clinical trial. *Pain* 48, 137-146.

Syrjala K.L., Donaldson G.W., Davis M.W., Kippes M.E., Carr J.E., 1995. Relaxation and imagery and cognitive-behavioral training reduce pain during cancer treatment: a controlled clinical trial. *Pain* 63, 189-198.

Sysko R., Walsh B.T., 2007. A systematic review of placebo response in studies of bipolar mania. *J Clin Psychiatry* 68, 1213-1217.

Tache Y., Garrick T., Raybould H., 1990. Central nervous system action of peptides to influence gastrointestinal motor function. *Gastroenterology* 98, 517-528.

Tache Y., Martinez V., Wang L., Million M., 2004a. CRF1 receptor signaling pathways are involved in stress-related alterations of colonic function and viscerosensitivity: implications for irritable bowel syndrome. *Br J Pharmacol* 141, 1321-1330.

Tache Y., Perdue M.H., 2004b. Role of peripheral CRF signalling pathways in stress-related alterations of gut motility and mucosal function. *Neurogastroenterol Motil* 16 Suppl 1, 137-142.

Tada H., Fujita M., Harris M., Tatewaki M., Nakagawa K., Yamamura T., Pappas T.N., Takahashi T., 2003. Neural mechanism of acupuncture-induced gastric relaxations in rats. *Dig Dis Sci* 48, 59-68.

Takahashi T., 2006. Acupuncture for functional gastrointestinal disorders. J *Gastroenterol* 41, 408-417.

Takahashi T., 2011. Mechanism of acupuncture on neuromodulation in the gut: A review. *Neuromodulation* 14, 8-12.

Talley N.J., 1994. Why do functional gastrointestinal disorders come and go? *Dig Dis Sci* 39, 673-677.

Tam K.C., Yiu H.H., 1975. The effect of acupuncture on essential hypertension. *Am J Chin Med* (Gard City N Y) 3, 369-375.

Tang Y.Y., Ma Y., Fan Y., Feng H., Wang J., Feng S., Lu Q., Hu B., Lin Y., Li J., Zhang Y., Wang Y., Zhou L., Fan M., 2009. Central and autonomic nervous system interaction is altered by short-term meditation. *Proc Natl Acad Sci U S A* 106, 8865-8870.

Taniguchi H., Imai K., Ludwig K., Takahashi T., 2012. Effects of acupuncture on stress-induced gastrointestinal dysmotility in conscious dogs. *Medical Acupuncture* 24, 43-49.

Tatewaki M., Harris M., Uemura K., Ueno T., Hoshino E., Shiotani A., Pappas T.N., Takahashi T., 2003. Dual effects of acupuncture on gastric motility in conscious rats. *Am J Physiol Regul Integr Comp Physiol* 285, R862-872.

Tatewaki M., Strickland C., Fukuda H., Tsuchida D., Hoshino E., Pappas T.N., Takahashi T., 2005. Effects of acupuncture on vasopressin-induced emesis in conscious dogs. *Am J Physiol Regul Integr Comp Physiol* 288, R401-408.

Taylor R.S., Brown A., Ebrahim S., Jolliffe J., Noorani H., Rees K., Skidmore B., Stone J.A., Thompson D.R., Oldridge N., 2004. Exercise-based rehabilitation for patients with coronary heart disease: systematic review and meta-analysis of randomized controlled trials. *Am J Med* 116, 682-692.

Taylor-Piliae R.E., Haskell W.L., 2007. Tai Chi exercise and stroke rehabilitation. *Top Stroke Rehabil* 14, 9-22.

Teasell R.W., McClure J.A., Walton D., Pretty J., Salter K., Meyer M., Sequeira K., Death B., 2010. A research synthesis of therapeutic interventions for whiplash-associated disorder (WAD): part 4 - noninvasive interventions for chronic WAD. *Pain Res Manag* 15, 313-322.

Teets R.Y., Dahmer S., Scott E., 2010. Integrative medicine approach to chronic pain. P*rim Care* 37, 407-421.

Teixeira M.Z., Guedes C.H., Barreto P.V., Martins M.A., 2010. The placebo effect and homeopathy. *Homeopathy* 99, 119-129.

Tekur P., Singphow C., Nagendra H.R., Raghuram N., 2008. Effect of short-term intensive yoga program on pain, functional disability and spinal flexibility in chronic low back pain: a randomized control study. *J Altern Complement Med* 14, 637-644.

Telles S., Gaur V., Balkrishna A., 2009. Effect of a yoga practice session and a yoga theory session on state anxiety. *Percept Mot Skills* 109, 924-930.

Telles S., Naveen V.K., Balkrishna A., Kumar S., 2010. Short term health impact of a yoga and diet change program on obesity. *Med Sci Monit* 16, CR35-40.

Telles S., Reddy S.K., Nagendra H.R., 2000. Oxygen consumption and respiration following two yoga relaxation techniques. *Appl Psychophysiol Biofeedback* 25, 221-227.

The-Henry-J-Kaiser-Family-Foundation, 2001. Prescription drug trends: a chartbook update. Publ no 3112. Menlo Park (CA): The Foundation, p. 45. www.kff.org.

Thorgrimsen L., Spector A., Wiles A., Orrell M., 2003. Aroma therapy for dementia. Cochrane Database Syst Rev, CD003150.

Tillisch K., 2006. Complementary and alternative medicine for functional gastrointestinal disorders. Gut 55, 593-596.

Toney G.M., Mifflin S.W., 2000. Sensory modalities conveyed in the hindlimb somatic afferent input to nucleus tractus solitarius. *J Appl Physiol* 88, 2062-2073.

Toth I., Neumann I.D., Slattery D.A., 2012. Central administration of oxytocin receptor ligands affects cued fear extinction in rats and mice in a timepoint-dependent manner. *Psychopharmacology* (Berl).

Tough E.A., White A.R., Cummings T.M., Richards S.H., Campbell J.L., 2009. Acupuncture and dry needling in the management of myofascial trigger point pain: a systematic review and meta-analysis of randomised controlled trials. *Eur J Pain* 13, 3-10.

Travagli R.A., Gillis R.A., Vicini S., 1992. Effects of thyrotropin-releasing hormone on neurons in rat dorsal motor nucleus of the vagus, in vitro. *Am J Physiol* 263, G508-517.

Tsatsoulis A., Fountoulakis S., 2006. The protective role of exercise on stress system dysregulation and comorbidities. *Ann N Y Acad Sci* 1083, 196-213.

Turk D.C., 2002. Clinical effectiveness and cost-effectiveness of treatments for patients with chronic pain. *Clin J Pain* 18, 355-365.

Turk D.C., Wilson H.D., Cahana A., 2011. Treatment of chronic non-cancer pain. *Lancet* 377, 2226-2235.

Uchino B.N., Cacioppo J.T., Kiecolt-Glaser J.K., 1996. The relationship between social support and physiological processes: a review with emphasis on underlying mechanisms and implications for health. *Psychol Bull* 119, 488-531.

Uebelacker L.A., Tremont G., Epstein-Lubow G., Gaudiano B.A., Gillette T., Kalibatseva Z., Miller I.W., 2010. Open trial of Vinyasa yoga for persistently depressed individuals: evidence of feasibility and acceptability. *Behav Modif* 34, 247-264.

Ulger O., Yagli N.V., 2010. Effects of yoga on the quality of life in cancer patients. *Complement Ther Clin Pract* 16, 60-63.

Uvanas-Moberg K., Arn I., Magnusson D., 2005. The psychobiology of emotion: the role of the oxytocinergic system. *Int J Behav Med* 12, 59-65.

Uvnas-Moberg K., 1996. Neuroendocrinology of the mother-child interaction. *Trends Endocrinol Metab* 7, 126-131.

Uvnas-Moberg K., 1997a. Oxytocin linked antistress effects--the relaxation and growth response. *Acta Physiol Scand Suppl* 640, 38-42.

Uvnas-Moberg K., 1997b. Physiological and endocrine effects of social contact. *Ann N Y Acad Sci* 807, 146-163.

Uvnas-Moberg K., 1998a. Antistress Pattern Induced by Oxytocin. *News Physiol* Sci 13, 22-25.

Uvnas-Moberg K., 1998b. Oxytocin may mediate the benefits of positive social interaction and emotions. *Psychoneuroendocrinology* 23, 819-835.

Uvnas-Moberg K., Ahlenius S., Hillegaart V., Alster P., 1994. High doses of oxytocin cause sedation and low doses cause an anxiolytic-like effect in male rats. *Pharmacol Biochem Behav* 49, 101-106.

Uvnas-Moberg K., Bjokstrand E., Hillegaart V., Ahlenius S., 1999. Oxytocin as a possible mediator of SSRI-induced antidepressant effects. *Psychopharmacology* (Berl) 142, 95-101.

Uvnas-Moberg K., Bruzelius G., Alster P., Lundeberg T., 1993. The antinociceptive effect of non-noxious sensory stimulation is mediated partly through oxytocinergic mechanisms. *Acta Physiol Scand* 149, 199-204.

Uvnas-Moberg K., Petersson M., 2005. Oxytocin, a mediator of anti-stress, well-being, social interaction, growth and healing. *Z Psychosom Med Psychother* 51, 57-80.

Valko M., Rhodes C.J., Moncol J., Izakovic M., Mazur M., 2006. Free radicals, metals and antioxidants in oxidative stress-induced cancer. *Chem Biol Interact* 160, 1-40.

van Middelkoop M., Rubinstein S.M., Verhagen A.P., Ostelo R.W., Koes B.W., van Tulder M.W., 2010. Exercise therapy for chronic nonspecific low-back pain. *Best Pract Res Clin Rheumatol* 24, 193-204.

Van Oosterwijck J., Nijs J., Meeus M., Lefever I., Huybrechts L., Lambrecht L., Paul L., 2010. Pain inhibition and postexertional malaise in myalgic encephalomyelitis/chronic fatigue syndrome: an experimental study. *J Intern Med* 268, 265-278.

Van Oosterwijck J., Nijs J., Meeus M., Van Loo M., Paul L., 2012. Lack of endogenous pain inhibition during exercise in people with chronic whiplash associated disorders: an experimental study. *J Pain* 13, 242-254.

Van Oudenhove L., Vandenberghe J., Demyttenaere K., Tack J., 2010. Psychosocial factors, psychiatric illness and functional gastrointestinal disorders: a historical perspective. *Digestion* 82, 201-210.

van Praag H., Shubert T., Zhao C., Gage F.H., 2005. Exercise enhances learning and hippocampal neurogenesis in aged mice. *J Neurosci* 25, 8680-8685.

Vase L., Robinson M.E., Verne G.N., Price D.D., 2005. Increased placebo analgesia over time in irritable bowel syndrome (IBS) patients is associated with desire and expectation but not endogenous opioid mechanisms. *Pain* 115, 338-347.

Vassallo M., Camilleri M., Phillips S.F., Brown M.L., Chapman N.J., Thomforde G.M., 1992. Transit through the proximal colon influences stool weight in the irritable bowel syndrome. *Gastroenterology* 102, 102-108.

Vaynman S., Gomez-Pinilla F., 2006. Revenge of the "sit": how lifestyle impacts neuronal and cognitive health through molecular systems that interface energy metabolism with neuronal plasticity. *J Neurosci Res* 84, 699-715.

Verbalis J.G., McCann M.J., McHale C.M., Stricker E.M., 1986. Oxytocin secretion in response to cholecystokinin and food: differentiation of nausea from satiety. *Science* 232, 1417-1419.

Verma S.K., Singh J., Khamesra R., Bordia A., 1993. Effect of ginger on platelet aggregation in man. *Indian J Med Res* 98, 240-242.

Vignozzi L., Filippi S., Luconi M., Morelli A., Mancina R., Marini M., Vannelli G.B., Granchi S., Orlando C., Gelmini S., Ledda F., Forti G., Maggi M., 2004. Oxytocin receptor is expressed in the penis and mediates an estrogen-dependent smooth muscle contractility. *Endocrinology* 145, 1823-1834.

Vita J.A., 2002. Nitric oxide-dependent vasodilation in human subjects. *Methods Enzymol* 359, 186-200.

Von Korff M., Wagner E.H., Dworkin S.F., Saunders K.W., 1991. Chronic pain and use of ambulatory health care. *Psychosom Med* 53, 61-79.

Vona M., Rossi A., Capodaglio P., Rizzo S., Servi P., De Marchi M., Cobelli F., 2004. Impact of physical training and detraining on endothelium-dependent vasodilation in patients with recent acute myocardial infarction. *Am Heart J* 147, 1039-1046.

Voss J.A., Good M., Yates B., Baun M.M., Thompson A., Hertzog M., 2004. Sedative music reduces anxiety and pain during chair rest after open-heart surgery. *Pain* 112, 197-203.

Wager T.D., Rilling J.K., Smith E.E., Sokolik A., Casey K.L., Davidson R.J., Kosslyn S.M., Rose R.M., Cohen J.D., 2004. Placebo-induced changes in FMRI in the anticipation and experience of pain. *Science* 303, 1162-1167.

Walsh B.T., Seidman S.N., Sysko R., Gould M., 2002. Placebo response in studies of major depression: variable, substantial, and growing. *Jama* 287, 1840-1847.

Wang H., Wessendorf M.W., 2002a. Mu- and delta-opioid receptor mRNAs are expressed in periaqueductal gray neurons projecting to the rostral ventromedial medulla. *Neuroscience* 109, 619-634.

Wang L., 2004. Clinical observation on acupuncture treatment in 35 cases of diabetic gastroparesis. *J Tradit Chin Med* 24, 163-165.

Wang S., 1997. Traumatic stress and attachment. *Acta Physiol Scand Suppl* 640, 164-169.

Wang S.M., Kain Z.N., 2001. Auricular acupuncture: a potential treatment for anxiety. *Anesth Analg* 92, 548-553.

Wang S.M., Kulkarni L., Dolev J., Kain Z.N., 2002b. Music and preoperative anxiety: a randomized, controlled study. *Anesth Analg* 94, 1489-1494, table of contents.

Wang T., Xie K., Lu B., 1995. Neurotrophins promote maturation of developing neuromuscular synapses. *J Neurosci* 15, 4796-4805.

Warshafsky S., Kamer R.S., Sivak S.L., 1993. Effect of garlic on total serum cholesterol. A meta-analysis. *Ann Intern Med* 119, 599-605.

Washabau R.J., Fudge M., Price W.J., Barone F.C., 1995. GABA receptors in the dorsal motor nucleus of the vagus influence feline lower esophageal sphincter and gastric function. *Brain Res Bull* 38, 587-594.

Weatherley-Jones E., Thompson E.A., Thomas K.J., 2004. The placebo-controlled trial as a test of complementary and alternative medicine: observations from research experience of individualised homeopathic treatment. *Homeopathy* 93, 186-189.

Weil A., 2011. The state of the integrative medicine in the U.S. and Western World. *Chin J Integr Med* 17, 6-10.

Welin L., Tibblin G., Svardsudd K., Tibblin B., Ander-Peciva S., Larsson B., Wilhelmsen L., 1985. Prospective study of social influences on mortality. The study of men born in 1913 and 1923. *Lancet* 1, 915-918.

Wessberg J., Olausson H., Fernstrom K.W., Vallbo A.B., 2003. Receptive field properties of unmyelinated tactile afferents in the human skin. *J Neurophysiol* 89, 1567-1575.

West J., Otte C., Geher K., Johnson J., Mohr D.C., 2004. Effects of Hatha yoga and African dance on perceived stress, affect, and salivary cortisol. *Ann Behav Med* 28, 114-118.

Westen D., Morrison K., 2001. A multidimensional meta-analysis of treatments for depression, panic, and generalized anxiety disorder: an empirical examination of the status of empirically supported therapies. *J Consult Clin Psychol* 69, 875-899.

Whary M., Peper R., Borkowski G., Lawrence W., Ferguson F., 1993. The effects of group housing on the research use of the laboratory rabbit. *Lab Anim* 27, 330-341.

White A., 2009. Western medical acupuncture: a definition. *Acupunct Med* 27, 33-35.

Whiteside A., Hansen S., Chaudhuri A., 2004. Exercise lowers pain threshold in chronic fatigue syndrome. *Pain* 109, 497-499.

Whorwell P., Prior A., Farragher E., 1984. Controlled trial of hypnotherapy in the treatment of severe refractory irritable bowel syndrome. *Lancet* 2, 1232-1234.

Whorwell P.J., 1990. Hypnotherapy for selected gastrointestinal disorders. *Dig Dis* 8, 223-225.

Wiklund I., Carlsberg J., Lund B., 1986. A double-blind, placebocontrolled clinical study on the effect of a standarized ginseng extract on psychomotor performance in healthy volunteers. *J Ethnopharmacol* 16, 15–22.

Wilkie D.J., Kampbell J., Cutshall S., Halabisky H., Harmon H., Johnson L.P., Weinacht L., Rake-Marona M., 2000. Effects of massage on pain intensity, analgesics and quality of life in patients with cancer pain: a pilot study of a randomized clinical trial conducted within hospice care delivery. *Hosp J* 15, 31-53.

Williams J.W., Jr., Mulrow C.D., Chiquette E., Noel P.H., Aguilar C., Cornell J., 2000. A systematic review of newer pharmacotherapies for depression in adults: evidence report summary. *Ann Intern Med* 132, 743-756.

Williams K.A., Petronis J., Smith D., Goodrich D., Wu J., Ravi N., Doyle E.J., Jr., Gregory Juckett R., Munoz Kolar M., Gross R., Steinberg L., 2005. Effect of Iyengar yoga therapy for chronic low back pain. *Pain* 115, 107-117.

Wilson L.A., Wayman C.P., Jackson V.M., 2009. Neuropeptide modulation of a lumbar spinal reflex: potential implications for female sexual function. *J Sex Med* 6, 947-957.

Windle R.J., Kershaw Y.M., Shanks N., Wood S.A., Lightman S.L., Ingram C.D., 2004. Oxytocin attenuates stress-induced c-fos mRNA expression in specific forebrain regions associated with modulation of hypothalamo-pituitary-adrenal activity. *J Neurosci* 24, 2974-2982.

Windle R.J., Shanks N., Lightman S.L., Ingram C.D., 1997. Central oxytocin administration reduces stress-induced corticosterone release and anxiety behavior in rats. *Endocrinology* 138, 2829-2834.

Witt D.M., Winslow J.T., Insel T.R., 1992. Enhanced social interactions in rats following chronic, centrally infused oxytocin. *Pharmacol Biochem Behav* 43, 855-861.

Wittig R.M., Crockford C., Lehmann J., Whitten P.L., Seyfarth R.M., Cheney D.L., 2008. Focused grooming networks and stress alleviation in wild female baboons. *Horm Behav* 54, 170-177.

Woody E.Z., Barnier A.J., McConkey K.M., 2005. Multiple hypnotizabilities: differentiating the building blocks of hypnotic response. *Psychol Assess* 17, 200-211.

Wsol A., Cudnoch-Je drzejewska A., Szczepanska-Sadowska E., Kowalewski S., Dobruch J., 2009. Central oxytocin modulation of acute stress-induced cardiovascular responses after myocardial infarction in the rat. *Stress* 12, 517-525.

Wu C.L., Doong M.L., Wang P.S., 2008. Involvement of cholecystokinin receptor in the inhibition of gastrointestinal motility by oxytocin in ovariectomized rats. *Eur J Pharmacol* 580, 407-415.

Wu J., Yeung A.S., Schnyer R., Wang Y., Mischoulon D., 2012. Acupuncture for depression: a review of clinical applications. *Can J Psychiatry* 57, 397-405.

Wu P., Fuller C., Liu X., Lee H.C., Fan B., Hoven C.W., Mandell D., Wade C., Kronenberg F., 2007. Use of complementary and alternative medicine among women with depression: results of a national survey. *Psychiatr Serv* 58, 349-356.

Yang C.H., Lee B.B., Jung H.S., Shim I., Roh P.U., Golden G.T., 2002. Effect of electroacupuncture on response to immobilization stress. *Pharmacol Biochem Behav* 72, 847-855.

Yang J., Yang Y., Chen J.M., Liu W.Y., Wang C.H., Lin B.C., 2007. Effect of oxytocin on acupuncture analgesia in the rat. *Neuropeptides* 41, 285-292.

Yau M.K., 2008. Tai Chi exercise and the improvement of health and well-being in older adults. *Med Sport Sci* 52, 155-165.

Yeh G.Y., Wayne P.M., Phillips R.S., 2008. T'ai Chi exercise in patients with chronic heart failure. *Med Sport Sci* 52, 195-208.

Yogendra J., Yogendra H.J., Ambardekar S., Lele R.D., Shetty S., Dave M., Husein N., 2004. Beneficial effects of yoga lifestyle on reversibility of ischaemic heart disease: caring heart project of International Board of Yoga. *J Assoc Physicians India* 52, 283-289.

Yoshida M., Takayanagi Y., Inoue K., Kimura T., Young L.J., Onaka T., Nishimori K., 2009. Evidence that oxytocin exerts anxiolytic effects via oxytocin receptor expressed in serotonergic neurons in mice. *J Neurosci* 29, 2259-2271.

Yoshimoto S., Babygirija R., Dobner A., Ludwig K., Takahashi T., 2012a. Anti-stress effects of transcutaneous electrical nerve stimulation (TENS) on colonic motility in rats. *Dig Dis Sci* 57, 1213-1221.

Yoshimoto S., Cerjak D., Babygirija R., Bulbul M., Ludwig K., Takahashi T., 2012b. Hypothalamic circuit regulating colonic transit following chronic stress in rats. *Stress* 15, 227-236.

Yu X., Fumoto M., Nakatani Y., Sekiyama T., Kikuchi H., Seki Y., Sato-Suzuki I., Arita H., 2011. Activation of the anterior prefrontal cortex and serotonergic system is associated with improvements in mood and EEG changes induced by Zen meditation practice in novices. *Int J Psychophysiol* 80, 103-111.

Zak P.J., Kurzban R., Matzner W.T., 2005. Oxytocin is associated with human trustworthiness. *Horm Behav* 48, 522-527.

Zeidan F., Grant J.A., Brown C.A., McHaffie J.G., Coghill R.C., 2012. Mindfulness meditation-related pain relief: evidence for unique brain mechanisms in the regulation of pain. Neurosci Lett 520, 165-173.

Zeki S., 2007. The neurobiology of love. *FEBS Lett* 581, 2575-2579.

Zhang K.R., Liu H.T., Zhang H.F., Zhang Q.J., Li Q.X., Yu Q.J., Guo W.Y., Wang H.C., Gao F., 2007. Long-term aerobic exercise protects the heart against ischemia/reperfusion injury via PI3 kinase-dependent and Akt-mediated mechanism. *Apoptosis* 12, 1579-1588.

Zheng J., Babygirija R., Bulbul M., Cerjak D., Ludwig K., Takahashi T., 2010. Hypothalamic oxytocin mediates adaptation mechanism against chronic stress in rats. *Am J Physiol Gastrointest Liver Physiol* 299, G946-953.

Zhou W., Longhurst J.C., 2012. Neuroendocrine mechanisms of acupuncture in the treatment of hypertension. *Evid Based Complement Alternat Med.*

Zubieta J.K., Stohler C.S., 2009. Neurobiological mechanisms of placebo responses. *Ann N Y Acad Sci* 1156, 198-210.

About the Author

Education

1977 Kobe University School of Medicine, Kobe, Japan.
1985 Graduate School of Hyogo College of Medicine, Nishinomiya, Japan.
1990 Postdoctoral Fellow, Division of Gastroenterology, University of Michigan. Ann Arbor, MI.

Professional Training and Employment

1985 Assistant Professor, Second Department of Surgery, Hyogo College of Medicine Nishinomiya, Japan.
1990 Vice president, Sadamitsu Hospital, Kakogawa, Japan.
1992 Research Investigator, Division of Gastroenterology University of Michigan, Ann Arbor, MI.
1996 Assistant Research Scientist, Division of Gastroenterology University of Michigan, Ann Arbor, MI.
2000 Associate Professor, Dept. of Surgery, Duke University, Durham, NC.
2007 Professor, Dept. of Surgery, Duke University, Durham, NC.
2008 Professor, Dept. of Surgery, Medical College of Wisconsin, Milwaukee, WI.
2013 Professor, Dept. of Surgery and Dept. of Neurology, Medical College of Wisconsin, Milwaukee, WI.

Research Interest

Dr. Takahashi's research interest is brain-gut axis, autonomic nervous system, hypothalamic circuit of stress response, and mechanism of acupuncture.

Home Page

http://www.mcw.edu/colorectalsurgery/Research/TakahashiStudy.htm#.T99J5Ji1nQM

http://kenkodojoclinictoku.wordpress.com/

http://kenkodojoclinic.wordpress.com/ (Japanese)

INDEX

A

C

I

J

K

L

M

N

O

P

Q

R

T

U

V

W

X

Y

Z